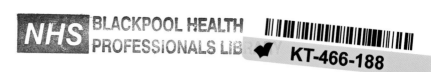
Rationing Medical Care on the Basis of Age

The moral dimensions

Eric Matthews

and

Elizabeth Russell

Foreword by
Kenneth Boyd

Radcliffe Publishing
Oxford • Seattle

Radcliffe Publishing Ltd
18 Marcham Road
Abingdon
Oxon OX14 1AA
United Kingdom

www.radcliffe-oxford.com
Electronic catalogue and worldwide online ordering facility.

British Library Cataloguing in Publication Data

A catalogue record for this book is available from the British Library.

ISBN-10: 1 84619 000 2
ISBN-13: 978 1 84619 000 1

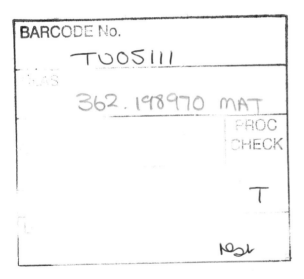
Typeset by Anne Joshua & Associates, Oxford
Printed and bound by TJ International Ltd, Padstow, Cornwall

Contents

Foreword

The idea that medical care can and should be rationed on the basis of age, however politically unpopular to articulate, has a long history in the hinterland of professional practice and popular consciousness. As this important and original book records, the claim that healthcare systems face a crisis as a result of the ageing of the population dates back at least to the 1930s, and since that time it has frequently resurfaced in discussion of the future of the British National Health Service. As in the case of many other social anxieties, however, the perception of a crisis has been more often uncritically entertained than carefully examined. The importance and originality of this book is that it now supplies a clearly argued ethical analysis of the complex medical, social and moral dimensions of this perceived crisis, leaving attentive readers in no doubt that the fundamental questions raised for society are indeed moral ones.

The subject of 'age-based rationing' has previously been discussed by a number of contemporary philosophers including, most prominently, Norman Daniels and Daniel Callahan. A particular merit of this book is its fair but critical analysis of the leading arguments of these and other philosophers in the light of the concepts of prudence, justice and solidarity and of the very different healthcare systems of North America and Northern Europe. By contextualising what for many readers have hitherto been rather abstract and, for some, rather alien debates, and by broadening their philosophical compass, the authors of this book have opened up significant new perspectives on many important issues which in practice confront politicians, managers, professionals, patients and the public today. Moreover, they have done this in a way that is highly accessible to a non-specialist readership.

Among the authors' most valuable contribution to contemporary debate on rationing is their analysis and application of the concept of solidarity. Their emphasis on the moral significance of solidarity reflects this book's origins in an interdisciplinary research project involving participants from Scotland, Iceland and Sweden, countries where public involvement in healthcare decision-making is particularly valued. But the authors' conclusion – that for healthcare rationing policies to be ethical they must not only in principle be based on morally relevant differences between people, but in practice be arrived at through informed and transparent public debate – is relevant not only to Britain and the Nordic countries, it is also an urgent and important message to all societies today which aspire to social justice.

This book does not come up with any easy answers to the question of how medical care can or should be rationed. It does however make very clear how and why easy answers in terms of age-based rationing can and should be resisted; and in offering a reasoned defence of appropriate rationing, it opens up the way to more mature debate and discussion of the issues involved. Eric Matthews and

Elizabeth Russell are to be congratulated on this major achievement, and this book is to be highly commended to everyone concerned with the future of healthcare.

Kenneth Boyd
Professor of Medical Ethics
College of Medicine and Veterinary Medicine
University of Edinburgh
July 2005

Preface

In 1998, an interdisciplinary and international research group based in the Centre for Philosophy, Technology and Society (CPTS) at the University of Aberdeen, Scotland, was funded by the Nuffield Trust to carry out a study of 'ethical and policy issues arising from the perceived impending crisis of old age'. The reference in the title was to the report *The Impending Crisis of Old Age: a challenge to ingenuity*, produced for the old Nuffield Provincial Hospitals Trust, the predecessor of the Nuffield Trust, in 1981 (Shegog, 1981). The 1981 report will be further discussed in Chapter 1, but essentially it was concerned with the possible problems created for the NHS by demographic projections of an increase in the proportion of retired people in the population. The aim of the CPTS group was to produce its own report (the present work) which would examine, 20 years and several changes of government policy later, whether this perception of crisis is still justified and, if so, what kind of crisis it is. As we shall see in the course of this work, various possibilities suggested themselves – a crisis of modern Western culture and its attitudes to ageing, a crisis of an increasingly technological and costly modern medicine, a crisis of the Welfare State, a crisis for individual doctors and nurses in dealing with their patients, to name but a few. We also aimed to see whether, whatever kind of crisis it was, it was peculiar to the NHS or whether, in some form or other, it might affect other kinds of system. But we came to the conclusion that in some ways our main problem was to decide on what kind of crisis it is: if that is not clear, it becomes impossible to consider how the crisis might be resolved.

But, as the wording of the report's title implies, there was a further aim: to examine the specifically *ethical* dimension to any possible crisis. CPTS existed to consider the ethical problems arising from technological and social developments. In this case, the project was based on the conviction that any problems for medical services created by an ageing population could not be satisfactorily analysed or resolved without taking into account fundamental ethical issues, of justice and rights, the duty to care for vulnerable people, respect for human dignity, and so on. The provision of medical care for any section of society cannot be simply a matter of economic efficiency or political acceptability, important though those considerations are. This is most obviously the case in the kinds of system of medical provision found in Britain and the Nordic countries represented in our group, in which, as we shall argue later, medical care is seen as a human right which society has a duty to provide for all its members. Konrad Obermann rightly says that 'Economic efficiency is defined by goals that are to be achieved and means that are necessary to it' (Obermann, 2000, p.221). If the goals of a system of medical provision are themselves ethical, then it follows that the system cannot be economically efficient unless it satisfies ethical standards.

If we are right about this, then if there is an 'impending crisis of ageing' for the NHS and similar systems, it must have an inescapably ethical character. The primary task of the CPTS group was thus to analyse the possible ethical problems which might arise for medical care as a result of the predicted shift in the age profile of society towards an increasing proportion of people over 65 (and indeed towards increasing proportions of still higher ages). Some people might question whether this could be a task for objective research. They see ethical questions as essentially non-rational – matters of emotional feeling or social convention. That is clearly not the view of ethics that underlies this work. Ethical values certainly do have an emotional basis: if we did not have certain human feelings, such as concern for others, we could not be said to be moral beings at all. But it does not follow that ethical judgements are *merely* expressions of emotion and so do not admit of rational discussion. Human beings want to live in a society in which the relations of one person to another are of a kind which both can find tolerable. That requires general acceptance of certain rules and standards governing how we should relate to each other. This acceptance of standards and values provides an area of common ground between the different parties to any disagreement about how to relate to each other in specific cases. Because of this common ground, debates about ethical issues cannot simply consist in expressions of personal feelings, since we have to aim to convince other people, if we can, that what we propose will produce a more tolerable situation in the light of standards which both parties share and of agreed facts about the existing position: that is the sense in which they proceed by reasoned argument. Research into ethical issues can thus take the form of a critical examination of the arguments used, including the factual information used in support of the ethical arguments. This in turn requires both a close analysis, of the kind familiar in moral philosophy, of the concepts used in the arguments and an evaluation of the evidence for the factual claims, of the kind found in the study of public health. In the case of our present topic, for instance, we need to be clear, on the one hand, what 'justice' means in relation to medical provision, what a claim to a 'right' involves in this context, whether we have special duties towards older people as such and, if so, what they are, and so on; and, on the other hand, in what way (if any) the facts of the current situation create problems of justice, rights and the care of older people.

Discussion of these problems, on this view, requires a mixture of abstract philosophical analysis and consideration of empirical data. From this point of view, the CPTS group was well constituted. There were two directors: Professor Eric Matthews, a philosopher with expertise in the philosophical analysis of issues in medical ethics, and long experience of collaboration with medical and related professionals and social scientists in discussion of such issues; and Professor Elizabeth Russell, Professor of Public Health, with a wealth of experience in empirical research in medical care. The other members of the group were all philosophers or theologians, but used to working in the medical context and in cooperation with medical and scientific colleagues. Two were colleagues from other institutions in Scotland – Rev Dr Kenneth Boyd, of the Medical Faculty in the University of Edinburgh, and Ms Sandra Marshall, of the Department of Philosophy in the University of Stirling. The other two represented the Nordic countries – Professor Mats Hansson, an ethicist working in the Department of Public Health and Caring Sciences, University of Uppsala, Sweden, and Professor Vilhjalmur Arnason, of the Department of Philosophy and Centre for Ethics, University of Iceland (and also a leading member of Icelandic Government Committees on issues in medical ethics). In addition to these standing members of the group, we were fortunate also to be able to call on the services of other colleagues from Aberdeen as relevant – notably Professor Ian Torrance and Dr

John Swinton of the Department of Divinity and Religious Studies and Professor Andrew Blaikie of the Department of Sociology. We were also fortunate to be allowed to use a paper independently prepared by a colleague from the Department of Public Health, Dr David Austin, in which he surveyed the historical development of the general principles of the NHS and of ideas about prioritisation, from the time of the Beveridge Report onwards. (An edited version of this paper constitutes Appendix 1.)

The mixed character of the project also determined its methodology. In this kind of work, the key thing is not so much the accumulation of data in itself, necessary though that is, as its discussion and analysis from an ethical point of view. In particular, the ethical literature is searched, not with the aim of extracting and expounding its findings, but as a stimulus to thought and argument. Thus, the choice of literature does not need to include all, or even most, of the publications in the relevant field, but can concentrate on those which the group found most illuminating and provocative. The central activity of the project was consequently that of discussion and debate which is the rough equivalent in the philosophical field of laboratory work in the sciences. It is a means by which different perspectives and insights can be presented and be subject to rational criticism by those with a different point of view. The aim is to arrive if possible at an eventual consensus, or at the very least, if consensus is unachievable, to set out as fairly as one can the various rationally justifiable points of view on the issue in question, thus at least clarifying the central questions to be answered.

The procedure that we adopted was that the two directors undertook the primary task of finding relevant readings in the literature of philosophical bioethics, public health and related fields. Because of the nature of the project, it was felt that using the normal bibliographical sources to search for material was not likely to be particularly fruitful. Rather, they started from work with which they were already familiar from their professional experience, and then explored further by following up references in these initial readings. Ideas, arguments and ways of formulating the questions suggested by these readings were critically and analytically discussed between the two lead researchers at their regular meetings in Aberdeen, with a view to seeing what conclusions might be drawn from them. At these meetings they were sometimes joined by the other Aberdeen colleagues mentioned above. The discussions and their conclusions were normally taped and also summarised in paper form for future reference. At intervals of roughly six months, a meeting of the wider international group in Aberdeen was arranged. The directors prepared for these meetings an account of their own discussions over the preceding months, emphasising what point they had reached, what problems and uncertainties they had encountered, and so on. The whole group could then, over the days of the meeting, take the discussion further, by adding their own individual and national perspectives. The international meetings were also taped and the tapes transcribed on paper. Contact was maintained between the international meetings, mostly by means of e-mail, so that further points could be made by colleagues outside Aberdeen. As is only to be expected, opinions on all sides changed and developed in the course of the project. At the end of the two-and-a-half years for which the project was funded, the two directors began the task of reflecting on and assimilating the conclusions, both of their own discussions and of those of the wider group, in order to distil them into the final report. Opinions continued to change even in this final period, and the report therefore went through several drafts before completion.

The present work is the ultimate outcome of all this discussion and reflection. The main body of the text was written by the two directors, using the transcripts of discussions between themselves and with the wider group; the directors alone, however, take full responsibility for what is contained in these chapters. After an examination of the history of the perception of impending crisis, of the costs of caring for older people and of the key ethical conceptions to be used in the analysis, there follow chapters on different interpretations of the alleged crisis. The conclusion we reach, in a nutshell, is that the idea that a crisis in the NHS is attributable to the ageing of the population has no substance, but that there are other sources of crisis for the NHS which will have a bearing on the care of older patients. Some of the implications of this are spelled out, not in the form of detailed policy suggestions, but in the form of ethical issues which will need to be taken account of by decision makers. The work concludes with three appendices by other authors, intended to widen the debate by placing it in more of a historical and international context. The first is an edited version of the paper by Dr David Austin referred to above. In the second, Professor Mats Hansson reflects from a Swedish point of view on justice and solidarity. In the third and final appendix, Professor Vilhjalmur Arnason examines the notion of justice in relation to the Nordic healthcare systems. The views expressed in these appendices are those of their authors as individuals, and sometimes differ from those expressed in the body of the text. The focus throughout the whole project is on systems of the same type as the NHS and the problems that they may face. We have considered other ways of delivering healthcare, especially wholly or partly market-based systems such as that prevailing in the US, but mainly for purposes of comparison. Apart from anything else, this counterbalances the potential distortions arising from the tendency, in most of the existing literature, to consider only the American situation. But our intention, to repeat, is not to offer detailed policy prescriptions for the NHS or any other system: rather, we have sought to analyse the ethical issues as an aid to those who must make practical decisions at different levels – politicians and policy analysts, health service managers, and clinicians in direct contact with patients. Our task will have been successfully completed if these decision makers are clearer about the ethical principles that underlie the present position in the UK, the nature of the choices they have to make, and the principles that they need to apply in making them.

Before concluding this Preface, we think it is useful to try to pre-empt some of the commonest possibilities for terminological confusion in this area. As well as helping to avoid misunderstandings in a purely verbal sense, this should help to make it clearer what we are attempting to do. (Our own discussions have often been bedevilled by questions of terminology in both these ways.) The first source of potential confusion is that the term 'health' is used very loosely and variably by different people in different contexts, sometimes with a precise intention and sometimes not. In the UK, the term 'National *Health* Service' (NHS) was coined at the inception of the Welfare State in the 1940s, because the aim of this particular component was indeed the health of the nation, at a time when medical technology was a shadow of its current self and when the modern distinction between the treatment of disease and the pursuit of positive health had not been promulgated. Now that circumstances have changed, however, failure to make such a distinction can be seriously misleading. We propose, therefore, to distinguish between '*medical*' services (concerned essentially with the treatment, by appropriately trained professionals, of disease, illness and injury) and '*health*' promotion (concerned with efforts to enhance positive health, including the prevention of disease). Since, in practice, only about 1% of the NHS's resources are spent on the latter, it is, in effect, a National *Medical* Service in our terms.

This leads on to a second point. There is anyway no uniformly used definition of health. The World Health Organization, as is well known, defined health as 'a state of complete mental, physical and social wellbeing'. But, apart from the fact that this can at best be regarded as an ideal, to which 'health' in the common-or-garden sense is only a very distant approximation, there is the fact that conceptions of what counts as 'complete wellbeing' vary from one individual and nation state to another, according to their differing beliefs and values. It is therefore almost incapable of a measurable common definition. One thing which does seem clear, however, is that positive mental, physical and social wellbeing (however defined) is promoted for the most part, not by what is done by medical technology, but rather by the environmental, social and political circumstances in which people live. This gives a further reason for distinguishing 'healthcare' from 'medical care'. In the present study, it is the latter which will be the prime focus because, as will emerge, it is the benefits and costs of technical medical services (in the sense just outlined) which are said to create the alleged 'crisis' with which we are concerned.

There is yet a further distinction to be made. Because older people are more likely to be physically or mentally frail than younger people, they have needs for care of a kind which fits neither under the rubric of 'health promotion' nor under that of 'medical services'. This is what is usually called 'social and personal' care: the provision of decent accommodation, help with daily tasks, and the like. The question of who provides which kind of care, how far the two sorts overlap, and how the agencies responsible relate to each other, is decided differently even within the UK, and certainly across the rest of Europe and the wider world. This means that the present study has had to concern itself with more than the NHS: the moral issues with which we are concerned often involve the overlap between 'medical' and 'social' services. It has therefore proved necessary at times to talk of 'care services' more generally.

Finally, as already stated, much of the relevant philosophical literature comes from the US, where there has until recently been no concept of a nationally provided service for either health or medicine, and where choices (although, crucially, within the limits of ability to pay) have been made by individuals at the level of consumption and not by governments at the level of provision. Most of this literature has used the term 'healthcare' or 'healthcare system', and so to be accurate it has been necessary to reflect this in the text.

In view of what has just been said, we have attempted to use the following terminology as consistently as possible in the text, except in direct quotations from the literature:

- 'Medical' care refers to medical interventions provided by medical professionals and services and aimed at treating illness, disease or injury, mainly through the NHS in the UK and comparable systems elsewhere.

- 'Health' refers to the subjective sense of wellbeing that is influenced by multiple components of individuals' lives and environments.
- 'Care' (without adjectival qualification) is used either to distinguish care from cure as the purpose of an intervention or, broadly, to encompass the services that try to meet the multiple needs of people that may cross agency boundaries, such as in the UK.

On the basis of our experience in discussing them during the study, we believe that these distinctions will be helpful rather than confusing. We hope that readers will agree.

Eric Matthews
Elizabeth Russell
July 2005

About the authors

Eric Matthews is Emeritus Professor of Philosophy and Honorary Research Professor of Medical and Psychiatric Ethics at the University of Aberdeen. He has a longstanding interest in medical ethics, in particular questions of resource allocation, and is the author of numerous publications and conference papers in the field. Until December 2004, he was a member of the MREC for Scotland, and is currently a member of the Clinical Ethics Committee of Grampian Health Board and of the Committee of the Royal College of Psychiatrists Philosophy Special Interest Group.

Elizabeth Russell is Emeritus Professor of Social Medicine at Aberdeen University. She has a longstanding interest in priority setting in healthcare, both the methods and the values underlying choices, and was medical adviser to the Scottish Health Economics Research Unit for 25 years and chair of the Scottish Health Services Research Committee for eight years. Her particular research interests are evaluation of medical care, ethics of healthcare rationing, measuring health outcomes and 'quality of life', inequalities in health and healthcare and consumer participation in health and medical care.

List of contributors

Professor Vilhjalmur Arnason
Professor of Philosophy
University of Iceland
Reykjavik
Iceland

Dr David Austin
Senior House Officer
Stobhill Hospital
Glasgow

Professor Mats Hansson
University of Uppsala
Uppsala
Sweden

Acknowledgements

The directors would like to express their gratitude for help with this study, above all to the Nuffield Trust for the funding which made it possible, but also to the colleagues already named above for their invaluable contributions to the discussions; to Dr David Austin for his kind permission to use his paper in our work; to the secretarial staff of the Departments of Philosophy and Public Health, University of Aberdeen, for their invaluable assistance at various stages in the project; and to the departments themselves for the use of their facilities.

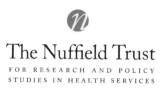

The Nuffield Trust

FOR RESEARCH AND POLICY
STUDIES IN HEALTH SERVICES

The Nuffield Trust is one of the leading independent health policy charitable trusts in the UK. It was established as the Nuffield Provincial Hospitals Trust in 1940 by Viscount Nuffield (William Morris), the founder of Morris Motors. In 1998 the Trustees agreed that the official name of the trust should more fully reflect the Trust's purposes and, in consultation with the Charity Commission, adopted the name The Nuffield Trust for Research and Policy Studies in Health Services, retaining 'The Nuffield Trust' as its working name.

The Nuffield Trust's mission is to promote independent analysis and informed debate on UK healthcare policy. The Nuffield Trust's purpose is to communicate evidence and encourage an exchange around developed or developing knowledge in order to illuminate recognised and emerging issues.

It achieves this through its principal activities:

- bringing together a wide national and international network of people involved in UK healthcare through a series of meetings, workshops and seminars
- commissioning research through its publications and grants programme to inform policy debate
- encouraging inter-disciplinary exchange between clinicians, legislators, academics, healthcare professionals and management, policy makers, industrialists and consumer groups
- supporting evidence-based health policy and practice
- sharing its knowledge in the home countries and internationally through partnerships and alliances.

To find out more, please refer to our website or contact:

The Nuffield Trust
59 New Cavendish St
London
W1G 7LP
Website: www.nuffieldtrust.org.uk
Email: mail@nuffieldtrust.org.uk
Tel: +44 (0)20 7631 8458
Fax: +44 (0)20 7631 8451

Charity number: 209201

List of Trustees

Chapter 1

Perceptions of crisis

Introduction

The idea that the population is ageing, and that this presents society with a crisis, is not new, and certainly did not first burst upon the scene with the Nuffield Report of 1981 referred to in the Preface. But it is interesting and illuminating to see both the similarities and the differences between various expressions of this idea, and in a report such as this we need to be clear *which* crisis we are talking about. To illustrate these differences, we shall consider two striking earlier examples of perceptions of a crisis of ageing, before comparing them with those of the 1981 report. We owe the first to our Aberdeen colleague, the sociologist Professor Andrew Blaikie, who helped us in our discussions. He points out in one of his studies of perceptions of ageing that:

> By the 1930s the demographic transition, largely as a result of falling fertility and infant mortality rates since the 1870s, prompted press speculation about a future Britain with deserted cities and idle factories while the spa towns were clogged up with pensioners in bath chairs . . . industrial retardation, spiralling welfare costs, a lack of economic enterprise, higher taxation . . . and a decline of 'creativity' and energy in the national psyche (Blaikie, 1999, p. 37).

The crisis described in this passage (let us call it for convenience the 'Blaikie scenario') seems then to have been largely seen as social, psychological and economic in character: it was thought of as one which would principally affect national productivity and energy. But it is significant that, in Blaikie's account, there is a reference to 'increased welfare costs' as well.

The second example comes a little later, during the Second World War. In this case, a crisis of ageing, slightly differently described, was seen primarily as creating problems for social insurance, in particular for the provision of retirement pensions. The Beveridge Report on *Social Insurance and Allied Services*, which helped to lay the foundations for the Welfare State, including the National Health Service (NHS), spoke of the need to take account of two facts in devising a plan for social insurance:

> The first of the two facts is the age constitution of the population, making it certain that persons past the age that is now regarded as the end of working life will be a much larger proportion of the whole community than at any time in the past. The second fact is the low reproduction rate of the British community today: unless this rate is raised very materially in the near future, a rapid and continuous decline of the population cannot be prevented. The first fact makes it

necessary to seek ways of postponing the age of retirement from work rather than hastening it (Beveridge Report, 1966, p. 8).

The assertion of the first of these two claims was based on demographic projections made at the time of its first publication in the 1940s, according to which 'in 1971, the children will be outnumbered by the possible pensioners' (Beveridge Report, 1966, p. 21). This state of affairs would be problematic, according to Beveridge, because of two of its implications:

> On the one hand, the provision made for old age must be satisfactory; otherwise great numbers may suffer. On the other hand, every shilling added to pension rates is extremely costly in total . . . . It is dangerous to be in any way lavish to old age, until adequate provision has been assured for all other vital needs, such as the prevention of disease and the adequate nutrition of the young (Beveridge Report, 1966, p. 92).

A little later on, the report speaks of the risk of imposing 'an intolerable financial burden on the community' by extravagant provision for its older members. The focus was on the cost of pensions above all, but the talk of 'provision . . . for all other vital needs' makes it clear that the welfare system as a whole is in view. The crisis in this case seems to be seen as one of additional *costs* for the system, which would in addition create a greater possibility of conflict between the old and the young. The report seems to be suggesting that the ageing of the population will force the community to decide how it can provide for the legitimate needs of the increased number of older members while avoiding excessively 'lavish' provision of welfare which would unjustly deprive younger people of some of their welfare needs, such as adequate nutrition. (There is also a reference to a potential conflict between the costs of providing for the specific needs of old age and those incurred in the prevention of disease, which is of course something that benefits all age groups, old as well as young.) The implication seems to be that in the circumstances envisaged, of increased numbers of older people and relatively fewer young people (because of the declining birth rate), even a fairly modest provision for older people might seem 'lavish', so that the resulting financial burden on the whole community would be 'intolerable'.

Thus, even in what is usually regarded as the foundation document of the British Welfare State and the NHS, there are forebodings of a crisis for that welfare system resulting from certain demographic facts, above all from the shift towards a society in which a greater proportion of the population than ever before were retired and in receipt of pensions. (For more on the Beveridge Report, specifically in relation to medical services, *see* Appendix 1.) The sense of foreboding was expressed again almost 40 years after the first publication of the Beveridge Report in the Nuffield Report of 1981 (Shegog, 1981), from which the title of the present work is derived: however, the focus of the anxiety this time was somewhat different.

In his Introduction to the report, ED Acheson describes how, in 1978, the Nuffield Trust held a special seminar to mark the thirtieth anniversary of the NHS, and to examine the problems that might face the service in the next 30 years. The main problem identified, he says:

is the marked increase in the numbers of very elderly and frail people which will occur in Britain in the next 20 years, and the consequent profound effects on society and its social and health services (Shegog, 1981, p. 1).

This 'marked increase' is quantified, and some of the 'profound effects' spelled out, in the next few pages. For example, Acheson quotes the prediction that:

there will be an increase in the numbers of people in England and Wales over the age of 75 greater than the present population of Liverpool by the end of the century. Moreover, it has been estimated [he goes on] that one in twenty of the population will suffer from incontinence (Shegog, 1981, p. 3).

This increase in the numbers of frail old people will be accompanied, Acheson argues, by a diminution in 'the number of able-bodied relatives available to share in the care of the elderly' (Shegog, 1981, p. 4).

Why should this be seen as creating a 'crisis'? In Acheson's view, the crisis would arise because of the vulnerability of older people and the greater costs of all kinds which this implies for their care:

This dramatic increase is in the age group which suffers from the greatest physical and mental disability and which requires six times more resources from the health services and twenty-six times more from the personal social services than the average for the rest of the adult population (Shegog, 1981, p. 7).

To a much greater extent than the earlier sources cited, then, Acheson focuses specifically on the 'health services' and the 'personal social services'. The frailty of old people is seen, not simply, as in the authors that Blaikie reports, as a cause of reduction of economic productivity for society as a whole, but as inevitably increasing the costs incurred in the provision of medical and personal care. These services, as he sees it, will come under strain because of the need to care for greatly increased numbers of precisely those people who are most in need of care. At the same time, more of this care will become the responsibility of publicly-provided services because of the reduction in the numbers of younger family members available to provide care at home. Acheson regards as unquestionable 'the right of the old to the best quality of care in hospital including where applicable the best diagnostic and therapeutic equipment' (Shegog, 1981, p. 18). This kind of care is usually expensive, so that to provide it for an increased number of older people will inevitably increase NHS costs, thus creating further strain on resources – an issue for public expenditure on which government concern had become focused since the dramatic increase in the price of oil in 1973.

But the crisis of resources seems, in Acheson's eyes at least, to be the most easily resoluble aspect of the problem: it can largely be solved, he thinks, by a more efficient and integrated use of existing resources and 'a strongly defined partnership with voluntary effort' (Shegog, 1981, p. 8). Much more difficult to overcome, in his view, will be another aspect to the predicted crisis. This lies in a cultural change in society's attitude to older people. In a more technological age, he argues, the particular skills of old people, based on a lifetime's experience, are valued less than younger people's ability to handle the new technologies. This devaluing of older people, he seems to be saying, has already led to a corresponding diminution in the status of geriatric care and of geriatricians, as compared with other hospital specialists. A consequence of this is 'alleged instances of elderly patients being given inadequate access to district general hospital facilities' (Shegog, 1981, p. 18): Acheson does not claim any clear evidence of the extent of such discrimination, but has the 'impression' that it is widespread.

Another contributor to the same volume, Vera Carstairs, presents the problem as entirely one of increased expenditure. Old people, she says, are high consumers of all health and social services, and she gives some examples:

> In addition to occupying most geriatric beds, the elderly occupy almost 40 per cent of all acute beds, about half the beds for mental illness and over 90 per cent of places in accommodation provided by or on behalf of local authorities. Recent government estimates have put the cost per head for health services as three times as great at 65–74, and six times as great at 75 and over, as at ages 16–64 (Shegog, 1981, p. 39).

If so, she goes on to say, then given 'that the present pattern of care continues, expenditure on health and personal social services for the elderly must increase . . .'. For Carstairs, then, the 'impending crisis' for the NHS will be one of spiralling upward costs, created by the increased numbers of over-65s and over-75s and the relatively greater costs of their medical and personal care: this problem will reach 'crisis' proportions.

The ethical nature of the 'crisis'

The sense of alarm in all three depictions of the near future is clear. The demographic projections on which this sense rests are the same in all cases (interestingly, despite the difference in the times at which they were made – a point to which we shall return). According to these projections, the numbers of people surviving to later and later ages is increasing, while at the same time the birth rate is declining. The inevitable result will be a shift in the traditional age balance of the population, with reduced numbers in the economically active segment (ages 16–64) and increased numbers of people past the present retirement age, and even above the age of 75. But the nature of the crisis described is subtly but importantly different in each case. In the 'Blaikie scenario', the product of a time before the development of the post-war Welfare State, it is seen as one affecting the socio-economic vitality of society as a whole. On the other hand, both the Beveridge and the Nuffield Reports take for granted the assumptions of the Welfare State, of an entitlement on the part of all citizens to taxation-funded social benefits, in particular to retirement pensions and to free access to a wide (and perhaps comprehensive) range of medical and personal services. For them, therefore, the 'impending crisis' is one specifically for the Welfare State as so conceived: the problem is one of providing these benefits at an adequate level for an increased number of people who are no longer economically productive, and from a reduced tax base. Acheson, in his contribution to the 1981 report, adds a further element, as we have seen: it is not just the changing proportions of old and young which will make things different, but a change in cultural perceptions of old and young – of the value placed on the respective qualities of older and younger people. Although Beveridge and Nuffield are alike in predicting a crisis of the Welfare State, however, they differ in the *aspects* of the welfare system on which they concentrate: Beveridge is mainly (though not exclusively) concerned with insurance and pensions, Nuffield entirely with medical and personal care. In the present work, we shall follow Nuffield in this respect: we have no contribution to make to the currently revived debates on the future of pensions, and shall focus only on the problems which are said to arise for the medical (and to a lesser extent the personal) care of an increasingly ageing population.

As was said earlier, it is interesting that the predictions of an ageing population were made at such different times. By the date of publication of the Nuffield Report, for instance, the projections made in the Beveridge Report should have *already* resulted in crisis, but the Nuffield Report still sees the crisis as 'impending'. This might make us suspicious of the fears expressed, including those expressed in 1981. Certainly, as we shall see in Chapter 2, some doubt has been expressed in the literature, on the basis of past experience, about whether an ageing population *necessarily* leads to increased costs for medical provision. Further discussion of this point belongs in Chapter 2, but for the moment we may say that it is never wise to be too cynical. Past experience is not always a good guide to future possibilities, and it may always be the case that the consequences of demography predicted may finally come about in the future. If so, it is prudent to think how one might deal with them *if* they come about (if they don't, then after all no harm will have been done). For this reason, we shall also accept without question that, whatever may have been the case with past predictions, this time the demographers have got their figures broadly right.

In all three of the examples cited, an important element in the perception of crisis is that the ageing of the population is seen as creating strains on the resources of society. There is a sense that the increasing numbers of retired people will become a *burden* on society, 'clogging up' towns with their bath-chairs, in danger of making 'lavish' demands on the welfare system and so increasing medical costs. But the welfare requirements of increased numbers of older people only create a 'strain' if the resources are not there to provide them. If medical care (to concentrate on that, since it is our main theme) is conceived as a marketable commodity, then, according to the ordinary laws of market economics, there can be no such strain. The resources needed in that case would be provided by consumers, and no one would be entitled to the commodity unless they were able to pay for it (i.e. to provide the necessary resources). If the increased numbers of older people could not provide the resources themselves (either from their present income or from previous contributions to insurance schemes), then they could not have the care in question: in other words, there would be no 'strain'. Strain arises only when we do not think of medical care in these market terms: when we think of it as a human right, to which all are entitled regardless of ability to pay, and for which the *state* must therefore provide the necessary resources. In other words, talk of a 'strain on resources' indicates once again that the impending crisis is one for a state-provided system – or, at least, a publicly-funded one. The Beveridge Report, as already quoted, speaks of the need for 'satisfactory provision' for old age in respect of pensions. As for specifically medical services, in the passage quoted above, Acheson speaks of the 'right of the old to the best quality of care in hospital including where applicable the best diagnostic and therapeutic equipment'. The crisis that we have to examine here, therefore, is a crisis of Welfare State structures like the NHS and the Nordic systems, and that is how we shall conceive of it from now on. In Chapter 3 and in Appendix 1, therefore, we shall examine the principles on which the NHS and similar systems are based.

It is here that ethical considerations become central. Talk of 'rights' to care necessarily places medical care in an ethical or moral context. It is connected with notions of justice and fairness, and we shall argue in Chapter 3 that the crisis arises particularly for systems like the NHS because the foundation principles of such systems are principles of social justice. If the crisis of ageing were purely financial, a problem of cost-containment without any moral implications, then we could solve them by purely technical means, as with any other area of government expenditure. For a start, we could, as Acheson and others have suggested, try what could be achieved by cutting out waste and inefficiency, by farming out relevant areas of activity to voluntary bodies, and so on. If this was insufficient, we could restrict the care available 'free at the point of access' on the NHS (perhaps confining it to what was most effective in achieving current social purposes, such as providing a healthy workforce) and leave it to individuals to pay for any other forms of care from their own pockets. Such a solution to the crisis of ageing would probably affect older people, and especially the less well off among them, more than most, but that would be a contingent result rather than part of the essence. The crisis, so conceived, would be a 'crisis of ageing' in the sense that it was *caused* by the ageing of the population, but it would *affect* the population at large. The 'rationing' of healthcare involved would apply to all, regardless of age, in the sense that the restrictions of medical provision would be based not on age as such but on factors, such as economic effectiveness, which are only contingently connected with age.

If such a solution is inconceivable in the NHS, it is precisely because the NHS has a moral foundation. Because it is meant to secure the *rights* of citizens to medical care, any form of rationing which is to be acceptable in the NHS must be one which does not deny anyone of any age any of their rights. So the 'crisis of ageing', even if it is interpreted as a crisis *caused by* the increased costs resulting from an ageing population, cannot be seen as purely financial, nor can its solution simply consist in reducing those costs. The 'strain' on resources will have to be seen as a *moral* strain. We shall need therefore to raise moral questions about whether costs can be reduced in particular respects without infringing anyone's right to medical care, and that will in turn involve some reflections of what our rights to medical care are – what they include and how far they extend. Hence, our inquiry in Chapter 3 will have to be also an examination of the whole notion of rights and justice in relation to medical care.

As soon as matters are expressed in this way, furthermore, a somewhat different conception of the 'crisis of ageing' comes into play. All citizens, including older ones, have (in the NHS and similar systems) rights to medical care appropriate to their needs. But since the system is funded out of general taxation, and the bulk of that taxation is paid by those of working age, could it not be that in the demographic circumstances envisaged it might be impossible to meet all the medical needs of the increased numbers of older people without doing an injustice to younger people – either through excessive increases in taxation, or through denying younger people some of their own medical needs? This thought is implicit in the Blaikie scenario's talk of increased taxation, in the Beveridge Report's references to excessively 'lavish' provision for older people at the expense of younger people, and in the implication in Acheson's discussion that younger people's resentment of the old might lead to the latter being refused access to some medical services. This would be a 'crisis of ageing', not simply in the sense that the ageing of the population caused an increased *drain* on resources, but also in the sense that it created new difficulties in *balancing* the use of resources as between young and old. Or, on a somewhat different interpretation (that of Daniel Callahan, to be considered in more detail in later chapters), it might be argued that the development of a technologically-based modern medicine has inflated *everyone's* notion of the medical care which is their 'right', but that this inflation has its most harmful expression in the demands of older people for expensive 'high-technology' medicine. In Callahan's view, as we shall see, the 'crisis of ageing' is in fact a crisis of modern culture, in its views both of the importance of medicine and of the significance of old age in human life.

On this conception, the crisis would not be one of justice in general, but one, as it is sometimes expressed, of 'intergenerational justice'. In the age distribution that has been found in our societies so far, the assumption is that this has not been a real problem. In a system like the NHS, it is the taxes paid by those of working age, as said above, which largely funds the provision of medical care for everyone, including both the young people themselves and those now retired from paid employment. This creates no problem of justice as long as the proportion of working-age people to retired people is large enough to provide what is perceived to be adequate medical care for both groups. But if the age balance of society changes sufficiently, with a smaller proportion of people of working age to carry the burden of funding the system, then, the argument is that there would be a 'crisis of ageing', in the sense of a problem of guaranteeing the rights of both older and younger people.

Some writers, such as Norman Daniels (to be considered in Chapter 5), would argue that talk of 'intergenerational justice' is a misleading way of thinking of the problems of ageing and healthcare, and would prefer to talk in terms of prudence over the lifespan. We shall, as just mentioned, critically examine Daniels's position later, but if it is rejected, then the 'crisis of ageing' could, it seems, be resolved only by means of a *fair* system of *age-based* rationing of medical care – one in which medical resources were allocated in ways which respected the rights of both old and young. Once again, this would raise fundamental ethical issues. Could any system of age-based rationing be regarded as 'fair'? To answer that question in turn requires us to think of rights to medical care in a more specific way than before: to ask whether (and if so why) rights to care might vary according to the age of the patients concerned, and whether we should think of different stages of life as having, so to speak, a different 'moral significance'. We can hardly avoid, in doing this, seeing the crisis of ageing, as Callahan suggests (and as is indeed implicit in some of Acheson's remarks quoted above), as in large part a crisis of modern Western culture.

In the light of what has just been said, we can try to explain the structure of the rest of the main part of this work. Chapter 2 will address the whole issue of the costs of caring for older people, examining the empirical literature on these questions, in order to provide a factual context for the ethical discussion. This chapter will thus be somewhat different in character from the rest, oriented more towards facts and their interpretation than to ethical issues as such, but the facts are necessary if the ethical analysis is to be realistic. Chapters 3 and 4 are in many ways the keystone of the work as a whole, and for that reason the most complex of all the chapters. They will provide the essential ethical foundation for the later chapters, by considering the NHS and similar systems as based on certain *moral* principles of solidarity and social justice. They will endeavour to clarify what those moral principles *mean*, as an essential part of understanding and criticising the different views of the nature and solution of the crisis of ageing to be considered.

Chapter 5 will then expound and critically analyse the views of the American philosopher Norman Daniels and, in particular, his proposal that talk of 'inter-generational justice' is misconceived, and that many of the problems of medical care for an ageing population are better understood in terms of what he calls a 'Prudential Lifespan Account'. In this chapter, as in Chapters 7 and 8, the method adopted will be first to expound the view in question in as fair and neutral a way as possible, and only then to engage in our own critical dissection of it and the conclusions to be drawn from that criticism. Chapter 6 will return to the discussion of general ethical questions. In view of Daniels's position, we have to re-examine the ethics of resource allocation in medicine, the concept of 'rationing' and connected issues. Then, in Chapters 7 and 8, we shall in the same way consider and subject to critical examination the idea that the crisis of ageing is fundamentally a crisis of modern technological medicine, as expounded in the recent writings of another distinguished American philosopher of medicine, Daniel Callahan, and as critically examined in the literature inspired by Callahan's writings. In Chapter 9, we shall attempt to draw together the threads of the earlier discussions and to present, based on them, our own conclusions about the issues considered. Chapter 10 summarises the implications of our arguments for policy making. The book as a whole closes with three appendices on historical and international perspectives on the problems.

Chapter 2

The costs of ageing

The ethical issues raised by the suggestions of limited resources need to be placed in the context of what actually seems to be happening currently in the provision of medical services for older people, and that is what we shall attempt to do in this chapter. In particular, it is worth devoting some space to the considerable literature suggesting that the predictions of greatly increased healthcare expenditure resulting from the ageing of the population are at the very least greatly exaggerated. If these suggestions are justified, it will put the predictions of an ethical crisis in a different light.

As already noted, the thrust of the Nuffield Report was towards improving care by better understanding and coordination of care across health, local government and voluntary sectors, so that older people would be supported in their time of failing capabilities and in the absence of enough of the younger generation to keep care within families. This thrust has continued in policy documents, culminating in the Sutherland Report of 1999 (Sutherland, 1999) although, as will be discussed later, practice has been extremely slow to follow policy.

By 1997 however, the position in respect of the needs and demands of older people had changed quite dramatically. What was not anticipated two decades earlier was the increase that would occur in older people's use of the acute hospital sector. The reasons for this have been multiple, but can be examined under three separate though interacting components. These are:

- 'need' – whether people have problems that it would be appropriate for medical care to try to help
- 'demand' – what citizens seek from medical services
- 'supply' – what is provided by the state, both in nature and volume.

All three are affected by changes over time that are most easily grouped as:

- population changes – the demography
- changes in the demand – created by needs, expectations and the likelihood of older people seeking care
- changes in the supply of services – in nature, volume and access.

Let us look at each of these in succession. (Much of the demographic and financial information in this chapter comes from the recent Wanless Report (Wanless, 2002) which was published on the same day as the April 2002 budget that announced a 50% increase in spending on the NHS.)

Population changes

The Nuffield Report noted that the main impact of older people would be the increase in numbers entering that age group rather than changes in their survival

(Carstairs in Shegog, 1981). Population predictions in 1981 were that in 2001 14.3% of the UK population would be aged 65 or more; in fact, that figure is about 16% (UK Health Statistics, 2001, Table 1.1). However, and crucially, the fact that life expectancy at aged 65 had begun to increase more rapidly was not recognised until the mid-1980s. From the first decade of the twentieth century until the mid-1970s, life expectancy at 65 increased by 1.7 years for men and 4.1 years for women (Carstairs in Shegog, 1981). In the 14 years from 1981 to 1995, life expectancy at 65 for men increased by the same amount, 1.7 years (to 14.7 years); and for women by only 1.4 years (to 18.3 years) (Wanless, 2001, para. 9.25). This rate of increase was faster for men, i.e. they are beginning to catch up with women, or women's rate of increase is beginning to slow down compared to that of men. So, improved survival in older people plus a continuing fall in birth rates means that the 'dependency ratio' – the ratio of children and pensioners to 16–64-year-olds – is rising. More than 80% of us in the UK wait until we are over 64 before we die (and thus, ironically, it is a good thing that old age is statistically more associated with old age than ever before!). As the 'baby boom' of the 1960s ages the absolute numbers of older people will continue to rise. Population predictions according to different but equally possible assumptions produce increases of between 3% and 13% (Wanless, 2001, para. 2.46). Thus, barring major disaster from infection or attack, there is no doubt that both the numbers and the proportion of older people in the population of the UK, and the Western world as a whole, will continue to increase at least for the next 20 years.

Changes in demand

The second source of a potential crisis for the NHS is an increase in demand for medical care. Obviously, given that the numbers of very old people are increasing quite dramatically, and they are in the age group most likely to be ill and to use medical care, then there will be a parallel increase in demand by them unless the average demand per capita falls. This could happen as a result of a fall in either their rates of illness or their expectations. In 1981 it was expected that disability in older people would be the prime source of need, and of pressure on the public sector. The evidence about patterns of disability is not easy to interpret because few longitudinal studies have been done that would observe how a cohort of people has aged at different times in the past. However, a comparison of two UK surveys that reported prevalence of disabled older people at home in 1985 and 1996/7 has shown some very relevant trends (Butterworth, 2001). Although the total numbers of all ages reporting some disability increased by an estimate of nearly 400 000, the estimated numbers in each of the three age bands over 64 fell by half a million in total. Note that these data do not include disabled people in residential homes, which house about 3% of the population aged 60 plus and who are there by definition of severe disability and need for continuous personal care. However, these numbers have not risen in recent years (Personal Social Services Statistics, 2002b). The greatest decline was in the age group 70–79. With regard to severity of disability:

* overall there was an increased rate in all levels except the most severe (categories 9/10)

- those aged 80 and above showed an estimated 50% decline in the rate of disabled in categories 9/10 but non-significant increases or no change in the milder categories
- the 70–79 age group showed a drop in all but the lowest level of severity
- the 60–69 age group showed an increase in the mid range (categories 5–8) but a decrease in both mild and severe levels.

Older people also reported a significant increase in related hospital attendance, in use of healthcare services at home and in day centres, and a significant decline in perceived unmet need.

These data were linked to aggregate data on living arrangements. Although the percentage of the population aged 65 or more who were disabled in private households declined markedly (from 43% in 1985 to 18.3% in 1997), the percentage in special needs housing increased markedly (from 4.6% to 16.8%) (Stearns and Butterworth, 2001).

Thus, very crudely, disability as defined in these studies may be expected to increase demand for long-term support with personal and nursing care, either at home or in residential non-hospital care, but not in the more severe categories nor attributable to the higher proportion of people in the very oldest category as was anticipated in the Nuffield Report. In the US, chronic disability among people aged 65 and over has declined faster in the 1990s than in the 1980s (Manton and Gu, 2001). Other evidence from the UK is that disability-free life expectancy at age 65 rose in 1976–91 from 11.0 years to 13.6 years for men and from 13.0 years to 16.9 years for women (Bebbington, 1998), which suggests that disability-free life expectancy is improving faster than total life expectancy – the desired 'compression of morbidity' into the last years of life (Fries, 1983). However, this estimate is not supported by more recent data, and is longer than the increase in self-reported 'free of limiting long-standing illness' that is used in the General Household Survey (Kelly and Baker, 2000; Wanless, 2001, para. 9.25).

In recent work, 'healthy life expectancy' (freedom from chronic illness that limits the ability to carry out normal tasks such as normal housework and shopping) has been distinguished from 'disability-free life expectancy', when someone is able to carry out their own personal care such as feeding, going to the toilet, bathing or being mobile (Sutherland, 1999, para. 2.22). Healthy life expectancy is a combination of self-reported factors in the General Household Survey for England and Wales (National Statistics, 2002), and includes 'limiting long-term illness', 'outdoor mobility' and 'activities of daily living'. 'Healthy life expectancy' has increased for men at 65 from 9.9 years in 1981 to 11.3 in 1995, and for women from 11.9 to 13.0 in the same time (Kelly and Baker, 2000). However, it is not as fast as the increase in life expectancy itself, implying that the number of unhealthy years of life is still increasing faster than the number of healthy years.

Based on the above pieces of data, Wanless concluded that 'while severe disability may decline, the number of minor health problems may increase as more of us live longer' (Wanless, 2001, para. 2.52). Thus the current assessment of the evidence suggests that disability *per se* is not the prime reason for an increased demand for healthcare in older people. Moreover, the extent of the change suggests that the perception of a crisis for the long-term care sector (Lancet editorial, 2003) as a result of increasing disability does not look like being fulfilled. This conclusion is supported by the Royal Commission on Long-Term Care (Sutherland, 1999) which drew on findings of the General Household Survey.

Demand for the acute care sector, and especially hospital care, is the source of most public and professional debate. In the absence of a more reliable measure, the use of services is taken as a rather poor proxy. Overall, the throughput of the NHS as reflected in volumes of episodes of care has risen continuously since the NHS began, as have its costs. However, the numbers of acute non-psychiatric hospital beds both available and used dropped by more than 30% in the decade 1990–2000 (UK Health Statistics, 2001, Table 5.2), partly because of much shorter lengths of hospital stay and partly because more care is given as outpatients or in primary care. About two-thirds of acute hospital beds are now used by people aged 65 or more compared to 40% in 1981 (Kendrick, personal communication, 2003; Carstairs in Shegog, 1981). This proportional change has arisen both from a fall in the rate of elective admissions, especially since 1995, at all older ages except those aged 85 and more, and from a marked rise in the rate of emergency admissions in the same age group (Kendrick and Conway, 2003). Hanlon *et al.,* (2000) looked at a cohort of 65–69-year-olds over 23 years and found no single risk factor (such as smoking or deprivation category) that was correlated with a rising rate of any kind of admission, yet the overall admission rate rose steadily. However, in absolute numbers this age group is tiny compared to the younger ages, and so for example the actual number of their emergency admissions is about the same as that of 15–44-year-olds although their rate is nearly ten times higher. Moreover, as stated above, the rate of elective admissions also rises with age, although in older people it began to fall in the mid-1990s, following the same fall that began in younger people a decade earlier (Kendrick, personal communication, 2003). These falls have been attributed to the increase in day care and suggest that older people are now better able to cope with day care as they are fitter and as techniques have been refined. What underlies these patterns? One factor is that people of all ages are postponing their illnesses to an older age just as they are postponing their deaths. So, undoubtedly, part of the increase in the volume of care of older patients, both absolutely and relative to younger patients, is that the burden of illness and dying has largely been transferred to the older group. Despite the survey data on mild disability, there is a lot of subjective evidence that people are indeed fitter for longer before they become ill or disabled. More than three-quarters of people aged 65 and over think that they are healthier than in their parents' time, and attribute it to better living standards, diet and healthcare (Cox *et al.,* 1993). In the US, higher levels of physical function in older age have been associated with prior healthier living (Brody, 1989). But another factor is that attitudes are changing. It is now socially unacceptable, except in the media, to describe someone under 75 as 'elderly'. 'Middle class' people, such as doctors, increasingly regard retirement as liberation, an opportunity to do the things, such as hill walking and canoeing, that the hectic pace of work no longer allows. Such positive attitudes are strongly related to control over one's housing and work, although the social class differentials in old age have become less because of state pensions (Williams, 1990). And, above all, older people themselves wish to be independent of the next generation and are more prepared to take risks than their children are to let them. 'Lock up your Grannie' is inverse paternalism which younger generations, slowly, are learning is unacceptable. The benefits of getting out and about are being recognised as outweighing the increased risk of accidents that may arise. Thus, as well as being healthier for longer, older people have higher expectations for their own fitness to participate and look after themselves. It is not yet clear that the attitudes of younger people to ageing have also undergone change. The Nuffield Report noted that the deterioration in society's attitudes to the aged was extremely serious; it reflected a loss of veneration because the scarcity factor had gone, and also because technology had replaced the sorts of skills that only the old and wise possessed (Shegog, 1981, p. 4). In the UK, there is another possible reason for a marked increase in the uptake of acute care by older people, and that is the fact that someone now 65 has lived all their adult life in the culture of the NHS with access to care that is perceived as a right and is free at the time of use.

Thus, although one might expect that if younger people are fitter and illness-free for longer then their demand for acute care might fall, and what one is seeing would be a transfer of need-related demand from younger people to older people because of overall improvement in health, the fact is that total demand at all ages is rising. Later in this chapter we shall look at the implications of this for costs of the NHS.

Changes in supply

The third factor that might create a sense of crisis in the NHS is a change in the supply of care, both in nature and in volume. New treatments since 1981 are many; they include the development of chemotherapy and the specialty of oncology, coronary artery surgery and, of course, hip replacement. Most of these will be used more by older people because they are more likely to have the underlying condition to be treated, and contribute to the trends described above. Also, some acute interventions have been shown to be just as, if not more, effective in older people: carotid artery surgery for stroke prevention yields greater absolute risk reduction in patients aged 75 and more than in younger ones (Alamowitch *et al.*, 2001). However, there have been many contemporaneous changes in the way in which healthcare and social care are accessed in the UK, and their effects are complex. Briefly, in 1993 there was a major change to separate long-term care from acute care and to place the former in the control of local government, which would act as a purchaser rather than provider of residential care (NHS and Community Care Act 1990). Within the NHS, the same Act created a purchaser/provider split within the NHS, the net effect of which was a rapid reduction in available surgical hospital beds and the consolidation of earlier policies to move psychiatric care into the community along with a more general move to primary care. Arguably, NHS productivity has also fallen in recent years because of shorter working hours, changes in terms and conditions of service for professional and support staff, and the introduction of audit, governance and other quality control procedures, for example arising from the Data Protection and Human Rights Acts, to which the system is now bound. All these changes have occurred against a backdrop of government debate about the need for the NHS to be more efficient and to prioritise its services so that those most in need are most likely to receive care (*see* Appendix 1). The background to this will be discussed further in the next chapter, but the point here is that the quality of and access to the NHS has been constantly on the government and media agenda for the last decade at least. The introduction by the new government in 1997 of politically attractive targets such as to reduce waiting lists and to have no one wait longer than two years for an elective procedure served to heighten the public debate, and gave a specific focus to complaints and concerns about access. A further issue more recently has been the introduction of pre-emptive clinical 'guidelines' and effective new treatments that cost money that many health authorities have been unable to find. This has fuelled concern about what the media have termed 'postcode prescribing', meaning geographical variation in supply, and usually of new 'high-tech' medicines or procedures.

Thus, whatever the reality of an increase in demand directly attributable to the ageing of the population, the NHS has been perceived to be in crisis because of its inability to meet demand in the acute sector, which is treating mainly older patients.

So, finally, let us look at long-term care and the implications of demographic changes. The Royal Commission on Long-Term Care in 1999 (Sutherland, 1999) set out 'to find a sustainable system of funding of long-term care for elderly people, both in their own homes and in other settings'. Its main conclusions (*see* Appendix 1) were that:

- one in five people in the UK who reach 65 are likely to need residential care
- collective provision or insurance by the state ('risk pooling') is required rather than personal/private insurance
- normal living and housing costs should be separated from the exceptional costs of personal care
- there should be a new body that brings together 'the many strands of long-term care under a single stewardship for the first time'.

It is interesting to compare these recommendations with the views of the Nuffield Working Group in 1981 (Shegog, 1981). The main ones were:

- a financial strategy that encourages freedom of choice
- no major increase in resources but a 'radical re-adjustment of existing resources' and a strong partnership with voluntary effort
- integration of accountability and planning within and between government departments and a single ministerial lead for social policy for the old
- a parallel integration at district level to create joint planning machinery and joint assessment of each individual
- an urgent review of cash benefits (including pensions) and subsidies and the working of the means test, and the creation of an interdepartmental group to create a single coherent financial strategy for the care of the old
- 'ungrudging and unashamed recognition of the part to be played by the voluntary and private sector in completing a comprehensive service to the old'.

At the time of writing, the financial strategy for pensioners in the UK has recently undergone a marked change. In Scotland, the devolved government has chosen to provide, as from July 2002, £125 million over the next two years for free personal care for all those in need of it (Community Care and Health (Scotland) Act 2002). Since 1993, joint assessment has been the responsibility of local government to arrange but there is still, and despite its clear reiteration in the Sutherland Report, no single body to look at long-term care or financial strategies for older (and disabled) people. The effect of the continuing split in responsibility and budgeting has been to prolong the potential for different priorities to be given to different components of the pathway of care. So, for example, one of the obvious effects of the 1993 removal of all long-term care from the NHS has been a return of delayed discharge (commonly called 'bed blocking'), i.e. hospital beds, usually in the acute sector, that are used inappropriately because the lack of temporary or long-term personal care support either at home or in residential care prevents someone's discharge from hospital.

Rather more progress has been made since 1981 on the involvement of the private sector in residential and nursing home care as part of the 1993 changes. By 1999, only 19% of residential places in the UK were provided by local government, 20% by voluntary homes, and the remaining 61% by the private sector (although there is considerable variation within the UK) (UK Health Statistics, 2001, Table 5.8). Recognition of the voluntary sector has focused largely on unpaid 'informal' care given by families and neighbours. The Sutherland Report accepted the conclusion of its researchers that, despite being influenced by demographic factors and living arrangements, the overall supply of informal care from children and spouses was unlikely to go down. However, in contrast to the Nuffield Report, it recommended strongly that statutory agencies must not depend on this when considering which older people should receive how much help.

There is very little published information about pressure of demand in the long-stay sector, perhaps because virtually all residential services and most domiciliary support are used by people aged 65 and more and therefore the scope for identifying age as a basis of discrimination is limited. However, it has recently been suggested that the NHS should sue local government for its failure to provide these services and thus create the back pressure effect on acute care that is said to account for about 6% or 4000 NHS beds in the UK (Public Accounts Committee, 2003).

Thus, although it appears that the impact of the ageing population may not be as dramatic in respect of 'burden of caring' as was anticipated 20 years ago, largely because people appear to be staying healthier and fitter for longer, it also appears that the increase in numbers of older people will continue to affect caring more than curing. The fact that the crisis in health circles has been perceived as being in the acute sector is interesting. Undoubtedly accusations of ageism have arisen within the NHS and mainly in the hospital non-emergency care sector, and the voluntary sector and media have not been slow to publish specific examples. However, this may be more to do with changes in the attitudes and expectations of older people, who are fitter for longer and want to be able to fend for themselves and do whatever they can to compress their own morbidity into as short a time as possible. They therefore seek and expect help on the basis of their need to stay active, rather than to stay alive.

It is of course the volume of care available, from whichever sector, relative to the increasing demand that is the nub of the practical dilemma that we shall go on to discuss in the rest of the book. If all needs and demands could be met, there would be no need to choose who should get care and who should not, whether by default or by choice, whether implicitly or explicitly. Before moving on, therefore, it is helpful to consider the current position about funding and the distribution of resources across different sectors and potential users of care in the UK.

Where does the money come from?

Contrary to much public perception, health spending in the UK is very largely publicly financed from general taxation (83%), not from personal payments that are earmarked for it. The remainder comes from the NHS element of National Insurance contributions (13%), charges paid by users (2%) and miscellaneous sources such as the increase in tobacco duty (Wellard, 2000). Healthcare in Canada, Australia and New Zealand is similarly funded mainly from taxation but these countries do not use social insurance (Wanless, 2001, Table 4.1). In much of the rest of Europe, although it is also largely publicly financed (average 75%), most comes from social insurance rather than general taxation (although the trend is towards increasing the proportion from general taxation) (Wanless, 2001, Table 4.1). Private healthcare in the UK currently accounts for about 17% of total health spending, which is low compared to the EU average of 25% and the Organisation for Economic Cooperation and Development (OECD) average of 26% (Wanless, 2001, para 3.21). Recent debate about alternative sources of funding UK healthcare has focused mainly on whether or not social insurance would be a preferred, and more effective, method. Social insurance systems depend more on employers' contributions but allow for individual users' contributions to increase according to their willingness to pay. In essence, the debate is seen as between increasing personal consumer choice through social insurance or using a central pool of public money to provide equitable access for all (Wanless, 2002; Irvine *et al.*, 2002). Current UK government policy is to continue to attempt to provide equitable access and to encourage involvement of the private sector not as user payments in the market place but as joint ventures with the government.

Where does the money go?

First, general taxation is distributed across nine main public service categories (HM Treasury, 2002, Appendix 1). Social Security (27.4%) is by far the biggest, health (14.5%) is next and education (12.4%) third. Other health and personal social services spend 3.5%. The remainder of the categories are not directly relevant to care. Within health, most of the £54 billion is spent on hospital and community health services (71%), while the Family Health Services (GPs, dentists, opticians and primary care prescribing) use about 23% (Wellard, 2000).

In the context of this report, it would be interesting to assess who uses general taxation spend, in particular which age groups, and whether older people use more than do younger people. This is not easy to do, as the categories of published data do not show uptake by age. However, a very broad picture can be seen in the analysis of relevant government public expenditure (Table 2.1). (Defence, Law and Order, Industry, Housing and Transport are not shown but together account for 21.94%.) It can be seen that, while it is likely that the combination of health and pensions expenditure makes older people the biggest age category of beneficiaries, the difference is not as wide as is often portrayed. It is also still true that average annual health expenditure per head is highest, at £2200 per year, both at birth and at age 85 or more (Wanless, 2001, Chart 2.6).

Table 2.1 Summary of UK taxation spending, 2000–01 estimated out-turn government expenditure on public services: how taxpayers' money is spent

Category	£ million	% of total budget
Education	46 000	12.37
Health	54 000	14.52
Other health and personal social services:		
Children	3000	0.81
Elderly people	6000	1.64
People with disability	3300	0.90
Social Security:		
Pensions benefits	38 700	10.39
Other benefits (unemployment etc.)	8500	2.30
Family benefits	9200	2.46
Disability benefits	11 250	3.02
Income support	17 900	4.80
Housing benefits	11 600	3.11

Also relevant is the expenditure of local government. Of about £13 billion in 1999–2000 (currently extrapolated from England only), nearly half (47%) is used for elderly clients and 37% for children including those with learning disability. Physical disability and mental health together use 12% (Personal Social Services, 2002a).

An analysis of NHS spending by age group in England and Wales (Seshmani and Gray, 2002) has confirmed that, between the mid-1980s and the mid-1990s, total spend actually fell in the over-64 group but rose in those aged 16–64, while costs per person rose at all ages but most slowly in the over-64s. This is in contrast to the position in other countries such as Japan, Canada and Australia, in all of which total spend on older age groups increased. However, when separate components of the NHS were examined, older ages had a larger increase in acute care costs than did the middle-aged groups. Thus it was concluded that the fall in the overall costs for older people was due primarily to a fall in their costs for non-acute hospital care. What cannot be said is why this happened, although it seems possible that it was in line with the policy to shift long-term care out of the NHS – whether or not older people are less in need of personal care than formerly. A Dutch analysis of the use of both acute and long-term care found that, between 1988 and 1994 in the Netherlands (which has the data to do this analysis), it appeared that the effect of new medical interventions was different in younger and older people (Polder et al., 2002). In younger people, there was a relative reduction over time in the cost of acute care but an increase in the number of people needing long-term care. In older people, there were more interventions per capita but a reduced growth rate for long-term care. In the US, the same differential effects of increased longevity on acute versus long-term care costs of Medicare was found but not the same pattern: acute care expenditures increased more slowly as age at death increased, whereas long-term care expenditure increased more rapidly (Spillman and Lubitz, 2000). The authors concluded that the effect of the increased numbers of older people was much greater than that of an increased rate of uptake per capita. In the UK, a Medical Research

Council longitudinal study found that higher weekly costs for personal and long-term care were strongly positively associated with living alone, being both mentally and physically frail, admission to continuing care, and death at the end of the episode, but not at all with age (McNamee *et al.*, 1999).

As some indication of the scale of the distribution across UK public sectors, the Sutherland Report presented estimated expenditure on long-term care (Sutherland, 1999, Table 2.2). It was estimated that, of a total of £11 billion at 1995/6 prices, 23% was spent by the NHS, 41% by the personal social services and 36% in the private sector.

A relevant question in the context of potential rationing or priority setting by age is who decides how it is spent. Given that most of the NHS budget comes from general taxation, decisions about how much goes to what or whom are taken at three broad levels, 'macro', 'meso', and 'micro' (Gillon, 1985):

1 Macro-allocation decisions allocate resources between government departments such as defence, transport, education and health, and between England and Wales, Scotland and Northern Ireland (*see* Levitt *et al.*, 1999, p. 103 for detail).
2 Meso-allocation decisions take place at two or three levels depending on the structure of the NHS at the time:
   – the allocation of resources to health authorities within a country
   – the allocation of resources between services or specialties within an area.
   Recent changes in the NHS Plan give power to primary care to control up to 75% of the NHS spend.
3 Micro-allocation decisions allocate resources between individual patients. These are almost invariably made by clinicians.

In practice, it is extremely difficult to know the criteria that are used for deciding who gets what and how much. Appendix 1 details successive NHS Acts and statutory documents since 1942 that have identified principles for the Welfare State and the NHS, such as that the latter is 'free at the point of use', and provides 'equality of access to healthcare'. At the macro level, government allocations from general taxation are the subject of the annual Budget statement and are derived from the annual Public Expenditure Survey Committee report that, in turn, is based on submissions from each department to the Treasury (Levitt *et al.*, 1999). At the meso level, attempts have been made since 1975 to distribute resources between health authorities according to 'need' as judged by the size and shape of the local population and its level of mortality (as a surrogate for the health effects of deprivation), and its existing use of hospital services (e.g., RAWP, 1976). Distribution between clinical services and sectors increasingly has become shaped by a plethora of national legislation and reports that recommend principles, priorities and plans that local health authorities are expected to follow, and against which their performance is likely to be assessed. However, only rarely is new money provided that is earmarked for any specific service, and none of these statements of priorities, such as naming cancer, heart disease and mental illness as the three most important clinical conditions to be tackled, identifies either the resource implications in financial terms or says what is to be given up to fund them. Moreover, the NHS Act makes it illegal (or is so interpreted by the Departments of Health) for any health authority to state publicly that a service will not be provided at all. And so, with some rare and innovative exceptions, choices of which services will be expanded and which contracted, or of who will not be treated, are both implicit at the health authority level and in practice left to clinicians to struggle with at the micro level because there is no precise allocation of money that they can identify and say 'we cannot afford to do x or y this month'.

It is undoubtedly true that part of the background to this report was, and is, the concern expressed by clinicians when confronted with such choices for the patient in front of them. In general, however, the debate about care arises not so much at the level of individual citizens and whether they receive help but rather at the level of local and national government priorities for how much of the available budget to devote to these services. In the following chapters, although government policy on both acute and long-term care is covered by many reports and Acts on the Welfare State, or the NHS and Community Care, the bulk of the evidence on any question of prioritising what older people have access to relative to others comes from acute medical care, and that is largely what we shall draw on for examples of the ethical issues that arise.

Chapter 3

The moral foundations of publicly-funded medical care

The meaning of 'moral foundation'

It has already been said in Chapter 1 that the NHS, and systems like it, is a system of medical provision which rests on an essentially moral foundation, and that that has a bearing on the way in which we have to understand the idea of a 'crisis of ageing'. But both these claims require clarification and justification, and that is what we shall attempt to provide in this chapter.

First, clarification – what exactly does it *mean* to say that the NHS rests on a 'moral foundation'? The briefest way to explain that is probably to say that, for the NHS, in the words of a slogan used by Norman Daniels, the American philosopher whose views on various aspects of our problem we shall be considering in this and the next two chapters, 'Healthcare is special' (cf. Daniels, 1985, Chapter 1). We shall be exploring what this means in more detail in a moment, but for now, by way of introduction, we can best explain it by saying that healthcare (by which, in this work, we mean principally medical care) is *not* to be thought of as a marketable commodity, like cars or refrigerators, but as a good of a significantly different kind. Goods that are appropriately supplied on a market basis are those whose goodness is entirely determined by the preferences of individual consumers, as expressed in the *demand* for those goods. A car is a good example: if no one wanted cars, then cars would have no value, and those which have the most value are those for which there is most demand (from those who can afford to pay for them). A car is a good thing for those who want one, but not everyone wants one. People may be said to *need* a car in specific circumstances, for example if they cannot do their job without one, but it would be nonsensical to describe a car as a universal 'human need'.

Medical care, or at least certain forms of it, is widely felt to be different from that. The difference is expressed, for instance, in the fact that human beings seem to find it natural to talk about a *right* to basic medical care, and think it morally wrong if for instance someone in great pain, or in danger of losing their life, is denied medical attention simply because they cannot afford to pay for it. Except in very special circumstances, it would by contrast not seem so natural to speak of a 'right' to have a car if one could not afford to pay for it. Medical care is felt to be a human need, a need of human beings as such, not just something that is needed by some human beings in some circumstances. Even in countries in which medical provision is largely organised on a market basis, there is usually some sense that emergency care at least must be available for those without the means to pay, usually on a charitable basis; and there is also, among some sections of the population in those countries, a feeling that something is amiss if the poor or unemployed are denied other forms of medical care because they are uninsured. It is this sense that morality and justice require medical care, or certain forms of it, to be provided to all, and therefore on a non-market basis, which is expressed in Daniels's slogan.

It is certainly historically true that the NHS was established primarily to give institutional expression to a moral right to medical care, and this is what is meant by saying that the NHS is supposed to have a 'moral foundation' – that provision of medical care is seen as a matter of social justice, rather than simply of a market in a particular kind of commodity. The Beveridge Report, in the spirit of national unity during the Second World War, proposed a scheme of social insurance as an essential part of post-war social reconstruction. The aim was to remove some of the obstacles to social progress, the 'five giants' that stood in the way of creating a better society. The 'giant' with which the report was primarily concerned was that of Want, that is, of poverty and all its consequences, but it also saw a need, as part of that concern, to tackle another 'giant', that of Disease. Disease made people unfit for gainful employment, so reducing their income. It was therefore the duty of a progressive state to seek as far as possible to *prevent* disease and, if that could not be done, to *cure* it. To this end, Beveridge saw as an essential part of any scheme of social insurance 'a comprehensive National Health Service', which would make available to every citizen 'whatever medical treatment he requires' and would ensure that this service 'be provided where needed without contribution conditions'. Significantly from our point of view, Beveridge declared that 'Restoration of a sick person to health is a duty of the state and the sick person'. (All quotations are from the Beveridge Report, 1966, pp. 158–9; for further discussion, *see* Appendix 1.) Ensuring that people are, as far as possible, fit for work is of course in the interests of society as a whole, but Beveridge puts more emphasis on the rights of individuals to be capable of providing for themselves and their families and so avoiding 'Want'. (It is worth noticing, however, that Beveridge also places a responsibility on individuals to do whatever is necessary to secure their own restoration to health; rights imply duties, as we shall see later.)

The Beveridge Report's proposals were given more concrete form in the 1944 White paper 'A National Health Service' (*see* Appendix 1) which outlined a scheme to provide 'the best medical and other facilities available' for everyone, regardless of their ability to pay. The resources for reducing ill health and promoting good health were not to be those of the individual, but of the *country*. Thus, the whole idea of a National Health Service has, from the outset, been based on the idea that the resources of the whole country, rather than those of individuals, ought to be used to provide medical care for every vulnerable citizen, on the basis simply of the individual's medical need, and be 'free at the point of use'. The whole language is again essentially *moral* in character, reinforcing the claim that the NHS rests on a moral foundation.

The next question that arises is that of the specific nature of that moral foundation. The Beveridge Report, as we have seen, implies that the state's duty to provide a national health service resulted from its duty to slay the giant of Want, by removing obstacles to individuals' capacity to work and so support themselves and their dependents. The White paper, on the other hand, clearly envisages a wider duty for the NHS, and this vision has persisted since the foundation of the service. Medical care is required, on this wider view, not simply to equip citizens for work, but to remove *all* forms of ill health. This is particularly relevant to our concerns, since it implies that a system like the NHS continues to have moral obligations to *retired* citizens, who no longer need to be fit for paid employment, and whose financial needs are meant to be met by the Beveridge Report's provisions for retirement pensions.

We thus have the picture of the NHS as a system that seeks to meet all the medical needs of all citizens, as a matter of moral right rather than of ability to pay. No clear limits are set to what can count as an acceptable medical need from the point of view of the system; and citizens are entitled to medical provision simply on moral grounds of humanity rather than of their particular characteristics as individuals (such as level of income, social status, gender, ethnicity, religious affiliation, etc.). Clearly such a system cannot be provided on a market basis, and the only alternative source of funding for it must be general taxation or compulsory insurance, which amounts, because of its compulsory nature, to a form of taxation. If, however, medical provision is to be genuinely independent of ability to pay, it seems to follow that the taxation which funds the system must itself be progressive: those who earn little cannot be expected to pay tax at the same rate as those who earn much, but must still be equally entitled to the medical care which these taxes support. Thus, a system with the kind of moral foundation that the NHS has must in effect be one where the medical needs of those with least income are subsidised by the taxes of those with greater incomes. By the same token, those who are employed and paying taxes will pay for the medical care of those who are unemployed, including those who have now grown too old to be employed (and those who are unable to work because of chronic sickness or disability). Furthermore, those who are healthiest, and thus least in need of medical care, will be paying in their taxes for those who are most in need.

The moral foundation of the NHS is thus not simply a conception of social justice, but one of what is often called *solidarity*, and it is indeed the latter conception which gives its particular flavour to the relevant idea of social justice. Many authors have pointed to the concept of solidarity as central to the idea of a Welfare State, and in particular to that component of the Welfare State which is called in Britain the National Health Service, and it is this concept which we need to explain more fully if we are to grasp the particular nature of any crisis of ageing which might confront the NHS. We can lead up to this concept by a quotation from the Beveridge Report:

> The prevention of want and the diminution and relief of disease – the special aim of the social services – are in fact a common interest of all citizens (Beveridge Report, 1966, p. 172).

The social insurance scheme and associated national health service which the Beveridge Report proposed was an expression of the sense that all citizens had certain 'common interests' as specified above – that all would be concerned for preventing want and diminishing and relieving disease of all others, whether or not they suffered want or disease themselves. It is this collective altruism which is the core meaning of the term 'solidarity'.

Hoffmeyr and McCarthy contrast social solidarity as a basis for resource distribution with utilitarianism, which aims above all for *efficiency* in the sense of achieving the 'greatest utility (or wellbeing) of the greatest number'. By contrast, they say, a 'solidaristic' approach takes into account values other than utility maximisation. It does this by using concepts such as 'sympathy' and 'commitment'. 'Sympathy', they say, 'concerns a direct interest in the utility of others', while commitment can be defined as 'a concern for others that does not affect one's own welfare'. Sympathy, according to these authors, is felt for 'groups to which the individual is closely connected' (such as family and friends), while commitment is to 'larger (and possibly anonymous) groups' (Hoffmeyr and McCarthy, 1994, pp. 226–9). In these terms, the kind of solidarity on which we are claiming the NHS is based derives from 'commitment' to the anonymous group of one's fellow citizens as a whole. It is the sense that all citizens, simply by virtue of being fellow citizens of the same state, have an interest in each other's wellbeing as well as their own. But the contrast with utilitarianism is that this commitment is not to the best *overall* balance of utility and disutility for society as a whole, which might well leave some individual members seriously disadvantaged. Rather, solidarity implies a concern that *each individual* in the group, including those who are personally unknown to ourselves, should have the best possible balance of utility and disutility for themselves. In a solidaristic system, we all pay our taxes so that those who are in greatest need should have access to most help, even if they are not ourselves or people to whom we are emotionally attached.

This is not irrational, provided we accept a certain conception of rationality. Rationality, on this conception, is not, as in more individualistic ways of thinking, a matter only of pursuing one's own best interests but also of doing what is necessary to promote the interests of others, even if that sometimes interferes with achieving what one would prefer for oneself. Although this has been expressed in terms of concern for fellow citizens, and in some forms of solidarity (e.g. nationalism) is *confined* to fellow members of the same community, in most forms it is extended to the whole of humanity, at least in principle. The duty to look after the interests of fellow citizens is held to derive from their *humanity*, and so, for example, to extend to all those originally from outside who may happen to become fellow citizens.

Another aspect of the idea of solidarity, with specific reference to medical care, is to be found in a Swedish Government Official Report of 1995 on prioritisation of medical services, which takes as one of its basic principles a 'principle of solidarity', which, when connected with the idea of justice, means that justice implies that 'resources should be committed to those fields . . . where needs are greatest' (Swedish Government Report, 1995, p. 20). (*See also* Appendix 2 – Mats Hansson's discussion of Scandinavian ideas of solidarity and justice.) If we have a duty to promote the wellbeing of all, then we have a duty to make sure that those whose wellbeing falls furthest short of acceptable levels are restored to such a level, i.e. to provide most for those who need most. Finally, we may quote some remarks of Nicholas Mays, Health Adviser to the Social Policy Branch of the New Zealand Treasury, from an article about potential threats to 'solidaristic' healthcare systems (Mays, 2000). Mays refers to arguments to the effect that:

> 'solidaristic', or universal, collective systems will face increasing challenges to their sustainability as rising demand for healthcare collides with the growing reluctance of the more affluent sections of the population to pay for services that will be mainly consumed by people other than themselves (Mays, 2000, p. 122).

The idea of solidarity implies that those best able to provide for their fellow citizens have the greatest duty to do so, even when they are not themselves in greatest need. In the words of the old Marxist slogan, 'From each according to his abilities, to each according to his needs' (a very neat summary of at any rate this aspect of solidarity). Thus we can say in summary that a solidaristic system of medical provision is one in which all members of a certain group (e.g. all citizens of a state) make contributions to the costs of the system, not simply in a spirit of individual self-interest, even enlightened self-interest, but out of a sense of commitment to those whose medical needs are greatest. 'Justice' and 'rights' in such a system have to be understood in connection with the idea of solidarity, of provision for those with the greatest need rather than those who make the greatest contribution.

Is this feeling anything more than a mere sentiment, or is it possible to construct a more rational argument for solidarity in this sense? To do so will require us first to get clear about concepts like justice and rights in a very general way. This will involve us necessarily in a certain amount of fairly abstract philosophical discussion, but we shall try to keep this to the indispensable minimum. We shall then consider a particular theory of justice and of the conditions of a just society, and in the next chapter ask whether it can be applied to the question of what constitutes a just system of medical provision, in particular one based on a solidaristic conception. At the end of the next chapter, we shall return to the question of a perceived crisis of ageing and see how the discussion of solidaristic justice may shed light on that.

What is it to have a right?

The concept of a 'right' in general is viewed with suspicion by many philosophers and political and legal theorists. To say that one person X has a 'right' to something seems to be something different from saying just that X *wants* that thing: it implies that X is somehow *morally entitled* to it. No matter how loudly someone may shout that they want higher pay, for example, their employer may quite legitimately, from a moral point of view, refuse to listen to their claims. They may then try to reinforce their claim by saying that they have a 'right' to higher pay: the use of the term 'right' is to put moral pressure on the hearer, to suggest that the hearer morally *ought* for some reason to grant the claim, that he or she has a *duty* to do so. The key phrase here is 'for some reason': claims that someone is morally obliged to do something require some kind of *justification*, in terms of accepted moral values. In this example, the claimants would have to appeal to moral values which are shared between them and the employer, and which would imply that they *deserve* higher pay. They might argue, for instance, that they deserve increased pay because they have worked harder, or undertaken more responsibility, or whatever. If this moral argument is valid, that is, if the moral values cited are genuinely shared by both employer and employees, then the employer is morally obliged to grant their claim: in other words, the employer has a *duty* to provide higher pay, and they have a *right* to it. This is the sense in which, as it is often put, rights and duties are correlative: to say that X has a right to something implies that someone else Y has a duty to ensure that X has it.

The type of duty involved may differ, as may the identity of Y, and this creates a distinction between different types of rights. One kind, often called 'liberty rights', comprises being able to do what one wants, unhindered by others, so that the corresponding duty is one on the part of those others *not* to hinder one in doing that thing. For instance, a right to free speech is a right not to be prevented (by state, or church, or majority pressure, or whatever) from saying what one wants to say. Another kind of right, often called a 'welfare right', is more relevant to our present topic. This is the right to *have* something, so that the duty on someone else is to *provide* one with that thing. For instance, a right to education is a right to be able to go to school, which implies a duty on someone (probably the state) to provide schools and teachers and to make them available to all those who have that right.

Sceptics about rights are normally not troubled by the idea of *legal* rights. After all, any system of laws can lay down what duties any person or institution within the relevant jurisdiction has towards any other person or institution, and so what rights the latter has within that system. It can specify precisely what duties and rights are, and under what conditions and in respect of whom they operate. Most importantly, it can back up rights and duties with sanctions: that is, it can enforce them by imposing penalties for failure to perform a duty or to satisfy a claim of right. In terms of legal rights, there can be no doubt that every citizen of the UK has a right to comprehensive medical provision, free at the point of use. However, problems arise, because it is claimed that this legal right ultimately rests on a *moral* or human right: the legal right was introduced because it was believed that the state has a *moral* duty to restore sick persons to health. To call it a moral duty is to imply that it has some foundation outside of and superior to any system of 'positive law', that it applies to human beings as such rather than because any particular legal system enjoins it, and that particular legal systems are therefore only morally acceptable because they conform to these universal moral concep-tions. It is here, for obvious reasons, that scepticism begins to arise. Surely, the doubters would say, there are no such universal human moral conceptions to which we can appeal as the basis for any idea that something is a *human* right as opposed to a right within a particular legal system. And, unless we invoke religious ideas, which are out of place in a purely secular discussion, there is anyway no universal authority to enforce moral duties and rights. Thus, some philosophers, like Jeremy Bentham, one of the leading figures in modern utilitarianism, have described the whole idea of (moral) rights as 'nonsense on stilts'.

This kind of scepticism is shared by many people other than philosophers like Bentham. For instance, the clinical geratologist John Grimley Evans, in the context of a King's Fund symposium on rationing in healthcare, makes the blunt statement:

> The notion, implicit in the writings of many ethicists, that there is an objective basis for a universal ethical system is a dangerous illusion (Grimley Evans, 1997, p. 116).

This statement, which sweepingly dismisses a whole central tradition of Western thought from Plato and Aristotle onwards, is made entirely dogmatically, without a shred of supporting argument. Grimley Evans clearly regards it as self-evident, which it certainly is not. But even if it is true, it would not preclude someone from arguing that, at least within the context of a particular culture, if not universally, it would make perfectly good sense to talk about moral (not just legal) rights to healthcare or to anything else. All that would need to be shown is that within that culture there are generally shared values on which such claims could rest. (To be fair to him, Grimley Evans (ibid.) acknowledges, for example, that within what he calls 'British national values' all citizens have an 'equal right . . . to live as they wish'. Thus some claims of right can be justified for him within the context of a particular local value system. We shall argue later ourselves that that is all that is required to justify the moral foundation of the NHS.)

If Daniels, or the founders of the NHS, are to maintain their position, they must counter such scepticism by showing that the right to medical care is something more than one guaranteed in some legal systems. It must be shown that the legal right is itself rooted in some more basic moral value, preferably universal, but at least widely shared within Western culture. The notions of 'rights' and of 'justice' go together – a just situation is one in which everyone gets their due, their rights, what they are entitled to or deserve. One way to make Daniels's case, therefore (and it is the one which Daniels himself adopts), would be to develop an acceptable theory of justice – one which would show that justice was necessary to the satisfactory ordering of any human society, and not merely something defined by the laws of particular societies. Daniels's favoured theory of justice is that expounded by possibly the most influential twentieth-century writer on the subject, the late John Rawls, above all in his monumental work *A Theory of Justice* (Rawls, 1973), but also in other books and in many articles. *A Theory of Justice* is undoubtedly the definitive statement of Rawls's position and of the arguments for it, and from the moment of its publication it has become one of the central reference points for discussions on the topic of justice, not only among academic philosophers, but also among politicians, social thinkers, economists and others. He has a fair claim to have represented, in its most systematic form, what 'justice' must mean in a fundamentally liberal society, such as Western European and North American nations consider themselves to be. Even his critics have tended to express their own alternative positions in his terms, in the sense of their degrees of similarity to, or difference from, Rawls. We can therefore, in a work like this, scarcely avoid coming to terms with what Rawls has to say. Fortunately, however, we do not need for our purposes to go into all the complex philosophical ramifications of Rawls's theory. We need only to examine those elements of it which are relevant to Daniels's attempt to apply it to justice in the field of medical care, and to our own subsequent critique of Daniels from a solidaristic point of view.

Rawls begins his account by claiming that 'The primary subject of the principles of social justice is the basic structure of society, the arrangement of major social institutions into one scheme of cooperation' (Rawls, 1973, p. 54). By an 'institution', as he explains a little further on, he means 'a public system of rules which defines offices and positions with their rights and duties, powers and immunities, and the like. These rules specify certain forms of action as permissible, others as forbidden; and they provide for certain penalties and defences, and so on, when violations occur' (Rawls, 1973, p. 55). He provides examples of 'institutions' (or, as he also calls them, 'practices') such as 'games and rituals, trials and parliaments, markets and systems of property' (ibid.). Rawls's underlying conception is that a human society is a set of interlocking rule-governed practices, and that we speak of a human society as 'good' when those practices, individually and as a whole, function in what we should consider a 'well-ordered' way. It is this 'well-ordered way of functioning', or at least a particular conception of good order, that we refer to by using the term 'just' or 'fair'. Hence, in one of his earliest essays, originally published in the *Philosophical Review* (1958), Rawls describes justice as 'a virtue of social institutions', and the principles of justice as 'formulating restrictions as to how practices may define positions and offices, and assign thereto powers and liabilities, rights and duties' (Rawls, 2000, p. 282). The principles of justice might be compared in some ways to the rules of the game, defining what is to count as an allowable move, what is to be regarded as a 'foul', and so on. But they differ from them in two important and related respects. First, and obviously, living together in society is not a mere 'game', but the serious core of our lives as human beings. And secondly, games have a particular predetermined aim as part of their definition, as the aim of playing football is to score more goals than the other side, or the aim of playing chess is to checkmate one's opponent. Living in society, according to Rawls, has no particular aim except to enable the individuals in society to achieve their own aims as completely as possible without preventing others from doing the same. As Rawls himself expresses it, his theory gives a 'procedural' account of justice – a set of rules for living together which does not depend on any particular conception of what 'the good life' consists of, and so enables different people with different conceptions of the good life to pursue their individual conceptions without interfering with others' pursuit of theirs. (This is, of course, why it is particularly appropriate to a liberal society.)

We can now examine in more detail both what Rawls means by 'justice' or 'fairness' and why he sees it as a virtue in a human social institution. Rawls thinks it useful to see institutions *as if* they had been set up by a group of rationally self-interested individuals. Each of these individuals would no doubt have his or her own conception of the good – of what he or she would regard as desirable in life. The principles of justice would then, on Rawls's view, be the rules which each member of such a group could reasonably accept as making only those concessions to the wishes of the other members as were necessary both to make social life together possible and to protect their own desires to the maximum possible extent. Only if such rules existed would it be rational for any of the members of the group to enter into the society. The implication of Rawls's argument is that what we mean by a 'fair' or 'just' social arrangement is one governed by such rules, in which everyone gets their due, but no more, and no one interferes, any more than is necessary for social living, with the activities of others. That such a society is the only kind that a rational individual could consent to join, in turn explains why justice or fairness is a virtue of societies.

This account, as Rawls says, has some significant resemblances to the idea of the 'social contract' as the basis for organised society, found in the classical political theorists of the seventeenth and eighteenth centuries, such as Hobbes, Locke and Rousseau. These theorists saw the acceptance of a rule-governed society, which limited people's natural freedom as individuals so as to ensure that no one person's freedom impinged on that of others, as the outcome of an agreement between people (the 'social contract') to abide by such rules as a way of avoiding the inconveniences of an antisocial 'state of nature'. Different thinkers conceived of the state of nature differently, and so saw different advantages in having an organised society. Hobbes, for instance, saw the state of nature as one of constant and unrestrained warfare between individuals and families, so that the social contract was to delegate everyone else's power over their own lives to the absolute authority of one individual (the 'sovereign') as the only way of keeping peace and so allowing civilised society. Locke and Rousseau put forward different conceptions both of the state of nature and of the aims of the social contract. But in somewhat the same way as all three thinkers, Rawls contends, we can think of our acceptance of rules of just conduct between individuals in a society or institution as if it were the outcome of a kind of contract between individuals to accept a set of rules which imposed the same restrictions on everyone's freedom in order to maximise the possibility that everyone would achieve as much as possible of their own good.

But there is one significant difference between Rawls and the old social contract theorists, and it is contained in the phrase 'as if'. Hobbes, Locke and Rousseau talk of their social contracts as at least possibly historical events – something which might have happened when human beings first moved from the wild state to living in settled communities. (There is some dispute among commentators about how literally this talk is meant to be taken, but certainly on the face of it they sound as if they are talking about the historical past.) Rawls, on the other hand, is quite clear that his 'social contract' is a *metaphor*, a 'thought-experiment' in which we imagine how human beings *might* behave *if* they were in a certain situation. The aim of the thought experiment is to make it clear what it is that makes certain rules rules of *justice* and why it is rational to obey such rules. Essentially, his point is that to count as rules of justice they must be *impartial* between individuals, giving no more importance to the interests or desires of one person than to those of others. For this reason, he elaborates the thought experiment. Those who formed the social contract should be imagined as meeting behind a 'veil of ignorance': that is, as all being equally ignorant of what their position was to be in the society which they were forming, and so ignorant of what their individual interests would be. In that situation, people could be genuinely impartial. However self-interested they were, it would be sensible for them to agree on a set of arrangements which meant that they would not be too disadvantaged *whatever* position they held, rather than to seek to gain advantages for any particular position, such as that of being rich, or holding political office, or being well educated. Given the mutability of human affairs, anyway, no one could guarantee that the position that one held at one time would continue to be held at others. Someone with political power at one time, for instance, might lose it and become simply a common citizen; it would be in his or her own interest, therefore, to make sure that common citizens were not too underprivileged by comparison with holders of political office.

So what basic arrangements would such self-interested, but ignorant, rational contractors agree to? First of all, Rawls argues, they would necessarily opt for an *equal distribution* of the basic goods of society (the goods which all members of society would see as essential for any life that they might want to lead).

> Since it is not reasonable for him [one of the contractors] to expect more than an equal share in the division of social goods, and since it is not rational for him to agree to less, the sensible thing for him to do is to acknowledge as the first principle of justice one requiring an equal distribution (Rawls, 1973, p. 150).

Thus, the first principle of justice is that justice implies equality in the distribution of at least basic goods. That in turn means equal *liberty* for everyone, including equality of opportunity, and also as far as possible (and compatible with other principles) an equal distribution of income and wealth.

However, it might be rational for someone operating from behind a veil of ignorance to agree that certain inequalities, at least in income and wealth, might be permissible, indeed might serve the goal of justice. Permissible inequalities would be those which could be shown to work to the benefit of the least advantaged members of the society. An example might be pay differentials which, by acting as an incentive to work harder or to take on more responsible positions, could increase the efficiency of the society and so produce more wealth even for the least well off. He would have nothing to gain by rejecting such inequalities, from which he would gain whether he was in an advantaged or a less advantaged position. This principle could not, however, justify inequalities of liberty or opportunity, since inequalities in these respects could not conceivably benefit the least well off. Lack of equality of opportunity would, on the contrary, remove the chance for the least advantaged to improve their situation. So any inequalities in power and income which were allowed would have to be attached to positions in society which were equally attainable by anyone, no matter what their starting point.

In summary, a just society or institution would, according to Rawls, be one which guaranteed equal liberty to everyone (so that no one was able to infringe the liberty of anyone else), equality of opportunity to achieve any position in the society (so that no one was prevented by the system from improving their own circumstances), and only such inequalities of income, wealth and power as could be justified by their beneficial effects for the least well off. And Rawls's argument about the 'veil of ignorance' is intended to show that it would be rational, in one's own enlightened self-interest, to value justice in this sense as a virtue in a society. Because it appeals only to the notion of rational self-interest, and is independent of particular conceptions of the good life, it can claim to have universal validity. It is not relative to the value conceptions of particular cultures, but only to a universal human interest in living as they want to live, while belonging to an organised society. The full and systematic development of these basic principles is lengthy and detailed, and would take us far away from our theme; but perhaps enough has been said to provide the background for understanding Norman Daniels's attempt to apply the Rawlsian conception to the field of medical care. We shall try to do this in the next chapter. Our method, as throughout this book, will be first to set out Daniels's position as clearly and fairly as possible and only then to comment on it. Nothing said in the exposition should therefore be taken as necessarily expressing our own views or as implying uncritical acceptance.

Chapter 4

Ethics and the 'crisis'

Norman Daniels and just healthcare

Daniels's writings on these themes comprise a number of books and articles, but his views on the general topic of justice in relation to medical care are most completely and systematically set out in his book *Just Health Care* (Daniels, 1985), which we shall mainly concentrate on in this chapter. (In his later book *Am I My Parents' Keeper?* (Daniels, 1988), which we shall examine more closely in the next chapter, he seeks to apply this general account to our theme of the problems of ageing.) Our interest here is in increasing our understanding of the solidaristic notion of justice implicit in the NHS and the Scandinavian systems, and its practical implications, by examining its similarities to and differences from Daniels's account. Daniels begins his book *Just Health Care* (Daniels, 1985) by reminding us that there are significant inequalities in the US healthcare system (on which, as an American, he naturally concentrates) which are correlated with race and class. It is the sense that this is morally wrong which gives rise to his slogan, 'Health care is special'. If medical care were simply regarded as a marketable commodity, inequalities in its distribution would raise no moral problems. In a market, no one has a right to anything unless they can afford to pay for it, and if someone does not have something they wish because they cannot afford it, then no injustice is done to them. But inequalities in the distribution of medical provision are seen by many even in the US as an injustice. Attempts to remedy this injustice by such programmes as Medicaid and Medicare, by Veterans Hospitals, by charitable provision, etc., mean that in the US what exists is a mixed, rather than a pure market, system.

However, Daniels recognises that it is not sufficient to *feel* this as an injustice. Some rational *argument* must be given to show that access to medical care is a right, denial of which constitutes an injustice. He attempts to provide such an argument, based on Rawls's theory of justice, while accepting that Rawls's view, in its original form, has no particular relevance to medical care. In particular, Rawls's list of 'primary goods at the disposition of society' includes only 'rights and liberties, powers and opportunities, income and wealth' (to which 'self-respect' is later added). Such other primary goods as 'health and vigour' are described as 'natural goods', in the sense that 'although their possession is influenced by the basic structure [of society], they are not so directly under its control' (*see* Rawls, 1973, p. 62). However, Daniels argues that health (or medical) care is a moral right because it is a fundamental human need, to which human beings as such are morally entitled. To call something a need, in this sense, Daniels contends, is to say that:

- it is objectively ascribable (that is, a need in this sense is different from what someone may *happen to think of as such*)
- it is objectively important (that is, is something which objectively plays some important role in human life) (Daniels, 1985, p. 25).

Daniels here refers to David Braybrooke's distinction (Braybrooke, 1968) between *course of life* needs (e.g food, shelter, clothing, rest, companionship, etc., which all human beings need at all times) and *adventitious* needs (things which are needed only in connection with particular projects on which a human being may happen to embark, as a student may need textbooks). It is *course of life* needs which most concern Daniels, since they are what is necessary 'to achieve or maintain *species-typical normal functioning*' (Daniels, 1985, p. 26) – the ability to live the kind of life which most members of our species can live. Sufficient food is clearly a need in that sense, since we cannot live in the way in which a member of our species normally can if we are deprived of adequate nutrition. But healthcare is equally such a need, since 'health', according to Daniels, *means* 'species-typical normal functioning' and healthcare is one of the things needed to maintain or restore such functioning when it is interfered with by the chance events of life. Hence, if medical care is not available, human beings faced with ill health have a reduced range of opportunity to live as most other human beings normally can.

Next we need to define more precisely what is meant by a 'range of opportunity to live as most other human beings normally can', or, to use Daniels's more concise phrase, a 'normal opportunity range'. Daniels does this in terms of 'reasonable life plans'. Human beings, he argues, can construct 'life plans', general views (which may be fairly vague) of the kind of life they would like to lead – the kind of career they would like to follow, the kinds of relationships they would like to form, the kinds of leisure activities which they enjoy, and so on. Different human beings may of course have different sorts of life plans, but we can distinguish in any given case between 'reasonable' and 'unreasonable' plans. A 'reasonable' life plan is one which could realistically be achieved, given normal human limitations and capacities, the particular inescapable limitations of the individual concerned, and the natural and social environment in which that individual lives. Thus, to have a life plan which included becoming a nuclear physicist would be 'reasonable' only for someone of sufficient intelligence and educability, living in a society which had developed scientifically to the level of nuclear physics, and which had educational institutions in which it was possible to study that science. For someone with serious learning difficulties, or who lived in a society that was scientifically undeveloped (and so did not have educational institutions of an appropriate kind), such a life plan would be 'unreasonable'. Some life plans, however, would be 'reasonable' for most human beings, since they would be achievable by the great majority of normally constituted human beings, with species-typical physical and mental capacities. So we can define the 'normal opportunity range' as 'the array of life plans reasonable persons in [a given society] are likely to construct for themselves' (Daniels, 1985, p. 33). (The restriction to a given society is necessary because what counts as reasonable even for a normally constituted human being may depend on the stage of cultural and social development of the society in which that human being lives.)

'Equality of opportunity' will then mean having an equal chance for everyone (at least in a given society) to achieve their reasonable life plan, where what is reasonable for any particular individual will in part depend on their individual capacities. (Not everyone, for instance, can become a nuclear physicist, and it is not a denial of equality of opportunity if those who lack the intellectual ability to benefit from the study of nuclear physics are denied access to such study.) Equality of opportunity in that sense can be denied in various ways. Someone with the intellectual ability to become a nuclear physicist, for instance, can be denied a university place because of poverty, or ethnic background, or gender. Social justice according to Rawls's theory would then require that such barriers of class, race or sex be removed.

But there is another way in which equality of opportunity can be denied, according to Daniels, and it is here that we come back to the theme of medical care. Someone for whom a particular life plan would otherwise have been reasonable may be prevented from achieving it because of disease or injury, and will thus be disadvantaged in comparison with others who have been lucky enough to avoid that misfortune. Someone who would otherwise have been able to become a professional footballer, for instance, may suffer a leg injury or a debilitating disease which, at least if left untreated, will deny them the possibility of pursuing that particular life plan, and will thus not have the same opportunities as others with the same basic physical capacities. Again, illness may interfere with the education necessary to pursue certain careers which would otherwise have formed part of perfectly reasonable life plans. Mental health problems may make it difficult for someone to form normal human relationships. And, clearly, most forms of illness may at least temporarily interfere with a person's ability to engage in normal human activities. If illness, disease or injury reduces equality of opportunity in this way, Daniels argues, then justice requires that these obstacles to equality should also be removed, and that in this case can be done only by medical treatment of some kind. This is the basis on which we can say that human beings have a 'right' to medical care. A just society, if he is correct, will be one in which there are arrangements in place to secure equality of opportunity for all members, and that will include arrangements to remove as far as possible the obstacles created by ill health, that is, to provide access to medical care for all. How far this is possible will depend on the state of medicine in the society in question. Where medical progress is limited, some obstacles cannot be removed, since no successful treatment exists. Thus, what is accessed by the 'right' to medical care will necessarily vary from one society to another. But no two members of the same society should be unequal in their rights of access to medical care.

This, in outline, is how Daniels seeks to fit a justification for claiming a right to healthcare into a Rawlsian account of social justice. But this account, as Daniels himself accepts, also sets limits to that right. 'Health care', he says, 'has normal functioning as its goal: it concentrates on a specific class of obvious disadvantages and tries to eliminate them' (Daniels, 1985, p. 46). We have a right, on this account, only to such medical care as is technically available and will restore us to the normal opportunity range for our society by removing some of the 'obvious' disadvantages created by disease or injury. But (and here our critical analysis begins) Daniels does not tell us in more specific terms what disadvantages are 'obvious' enough to count, although he does say on the same page that he is 'not committed to the futile goal of eliminating or "levelling" all natural differences between persons'. This is only one of a number of obscurities in Daniels's argument. It is worth exploring these obscurities further, since that will help us to see what is useful and what is not so useful in Daniels's position from the point of view of clarifying the moral basis of the NHS.

Daniels attempts to relate a right to medical care to Rawls's theory of justice by means of the notion of 'equality of opportunity'. Denial of equality of opportunity, in some sense of that term, seems to be *prima facie* unjust, so that it will be a characteristic of a just society that it ensures that the conditions for achieving equality in this respect are in place. But what these conditions *are* will depend on what we mean by 'opportunity'. What Daniels means by this term seems to be significantly different from what Rawls means. Rawls speaks, as we have seen, of certain primary goods at the disposition of society – rights and liberties, powers and opportunities, income and wealth – as relevant to justice. Equality in respect of these must be built into the arrangements of a just society, because they will secure the ability of each member to achieve their own good, no matter what their conception of the good may be, and to have access to positions of power and wealth in the society. In other words, these goods are 'procedural', rather than related to an individual's particular substantial conceptions of what the good life might consist of. Rawls, as we have also seen, places health in a different category, as something that cannot be directly provided by society (although, as he implies, social arrangements may indirectly contribute to health). Health is precisely a substantial good, although one which most sane individuals would want. In that sense, equality of opportunity is equality in primary social goods which would enable anyone *who wanted to* to have an equal possibility of pursuing such substantial goods as health (for instance, sufficient equality of income would enable everyone who wanted health to be able to pay for adequate medical care). Rawls's account in this way specifically rules out a 'right to healthcare' in the sense of a right of access to medical care free of charge. All that Rawls requires in a just society is sufficient equality of income to allow people access to whatever goods they pursue, which may well include medical care.

Daniels gives the appearance of a closer link to Rawls's theory in part because of his definition of 'health' in terms of 'species-specific normal functioning'. But this creates difficulties in itself. What, for instance, is meant by 'normal' in this case? Does it mean something value-neutral, such as 'usual' or 'average'? Most human beings can walk unaided, breathe without difficulty, digest their food properly (most of the time), see and hear, and so on. Some cannot do these things, or cannot do them as well as the majority, either because of disease or injury, or because of genetic factors, or indeed (and here we come closer to our theme) because of old age. If we say that everyone ought to have access to medical care which would make them closer to normal (average) functioning, then does that imply that everything which creates an obstacle to such functioning ought to be treated free of charge? After all, why should one way of deviating from the normal deserve medical treatment, but not all? Why should a young person who through injury is unable, say, to do the things which most human beings can do deserve treatment for her injury, while an old person who is similarly disabled, but by the frailties of her age, not have such a right? To extend the right to medical care in that way, however, would expose Daniels to another sort of objection, which is very relevant to our topic here. Daniels himself considers this objection, one that was raised by Charles Fried to the whole notion of a right to healthcare based on fair equality of opportunity. Fried (Fried, 1978) argues that to concede rights to healthcare on this basis would be too *expensive*, because it would increase costs by increasing demand. Daniels responds to this objection, interestingly, by arguing that his model in fact *excludes* some of the costs which bothered Fried, such as that of retarding the effects of normal ageing. His model does not imply that our healthcare rights extend to such anti-ageing treatment, since that would not be correcting a departure from our normal species functioning. He does concede, however, that his 'account of needs at best reduces but does not eliminate Fried's worry' (Daniels, 1985, p. 53). His reply here, however, implies that 'normal species functioning' does not mean simply 'how most people function', but means something like 'what is in accordance with the natural order of things'. Thus, it is 'natural' for human physical powers to decline with old age, so that the frailties of old age, which are so at variance with the characteristics of most human beings, are nevertheless part of normal species functioning. Then, however, the question arises: why should we accept something just because it is 'natural'? It is natural, in accordance with laws of nature, for someone who is infected by a certain virus to develop a fever: medicine seeks to treat that fever. So why is it not part of medicine's duty to try to correct the equally natural effects of ageing? There may be arguments to show that these two cases are different, but Daniels does not supply them. (We shall return to this point in the next chapter, when we consider Daniels's views specifically on just provision for old age.)

The root of the problem in Daniels's position seems to lie in his attempt to fit the right to medical care into a particular conception of justice as consisting of equality of opportunity for employment and office. It certainly seems to be true (as the Beveridge Report implies) that *one* reason why we value medical care is that it removes obstacles to employment and thus to income. But this cannot be the sole basis for asserting a right to medical care. Ill health is not, for one thing, always a barrier to employment. With determination, and with provision of appropriate employment opportunities, even those who are seriously disabled can often find employment without treatment of their disability. And even if that is not possible, it would be just as rational to provide those who are ill or disabled with an income which could enable them to provide medical care for themselves *if they wished it*, as to provide free state-aided medical care for all, even those who are bursting with health. More important still, however, is another consideration. The provision of equality of opportunities for employment is surely not the main reason why we value either health or the medical care that may maintain or restore it. Health is a good thing because it is a necessary condition for many other things which are part of what would be regarded as a desirable life: most people would say that it is better to be free of excessive pain, to avoid premature death, not to be incapacitated, in other words, to be healthy than it is to be unhealthy, whether or not it affects one's 'opportunities' for achieving social position or wealth. These reasons for valuing health are as relevant to retired people as to those of working age. But this does not, in itself and without further argument, seem to provide any justification for regarding access to medical care as a 'right', in the sense of something which ought to be provided for the individual citizen by the state and free at the point of use. It is significant that Daniels himself accepts that 'National health insurance is not an immediate consequence of asserting a right to healthcare' (Daniels, 1985, p. 9).

Equality of opportunity vs 'solidarity'

A Rawlsian account of justice, then, will not, at least on its own, provide the theoretical foundation for the moral status of the NHS. In order to do this, we must first go back to the concept of 'need', and of medical care as a need, and interpret it in a sense which does not relate it to 'species-specific normal functioning'. One of the present authors has proposed one way of trying to do this (Matthews, 1998). Daniels attempts to define need in objective biological terms. Course of life needs are what is necessary 'to achieve or maintain *species-typical normal functioning*' (Daniels, 1985, p. 26), where what counts as 'normal' functioning is supposed to be an objective, value-neutral, fact about our species. Furthermore, he identifies normal functioning in this sense with health, and deviations from it as illness. Medical care is then care that is needed to restore or maintain health. But there are several difficulties with these definitions. One is whether one can define normal functioning, or health, in such a value-neutral way. There seems to be no contradiction in saying, for instance, that a whole population might be sick (unwell, ill). If being healthy just meant being like most people, there would surely be some logical difficulty in saying that. We can say such things because we define 'normality' rather in terms of certain *norms* of how things *ought* to be, that is, in evaluative terms. Furthermore, if it were not so, then it is hard to see how one could validly derive such evaluative conclusions as 'Someone has a *duty* to provide medical care' from such premises. Why should there be any duty to make sure that everyone can do what most people can do? And what about the use of medical care to *improve* on what is naturally possible?

However, a different concept of 'need' is possible, one explicitly defined in terms of moral values rather than of biological facts. Matthews offers such a different concept of 'need'. A need in his sense is a good 'to which human beings as such [are] morally entitled, that is, a life without these goods would not be worthy of human beings' (Matthews, 1998, p. 157). A number of objections could be raised to this account. First, one of the apparent virtues of Daniels's definition is that it seems to rest on objective facts, and so to transcend any cultural relativism over values. In this sense, it would ground a right to medical care in any human culture whatsoever. Matthews's definition, by contrast, appeals to the vague notion of 'a life worthy of human beings', which seems clearly relative to a particular culture's conception of what is so worthy. At most, therefore, it could justify a claim of a right to medical care only to those who shared that cultural conception. On the other hand, just because it is allegedly objective, as we have seen, Daniels's definition cannot logically justify any evaluative claims about rights and duties. As David Hume pointed out, we cannot deduce an 'ought' from an 'is', a value judgement from a factual statement. As for the problem of relativism, if we remember that all our discussion is carried on within the frames of reference of Western liberal culture, that should not be such a difficulty. If we can show that, by Western liberal norms, there is a right to medical care, then that would be enough to provide a moral foundation for the NHS, a system which operates within a Western liberal society.

If we confine ourselves to our own society in this way, we could probably say that most people in our society would think that what is required (medically speaking) to make a person's life 'worthy of a human being' is:

- treatment aimed at enabling the person in question to reach the normal lifespan
- treatment to relieve undue and unchosen pain and distress
- treatment to put right disabilities.

All of these terms are in need of further definition and elaboration, but they are at least more precise and specific than the term 'worthy of a human being'. These could then be regarded as the basic medical *needs*. If we then say that human beings have a right to what is required for a decent life, we could conclude that they have a right to the provision of these basic medical needs. Nothing is said here about the thorny question of whether one sort of medical need has a moral *priority* over any other, which is the heart of the issue of so-called 'rationing' of medical care, which we shall return to later. All that is claimed here is that this account of the right to medical care is both wider in extent than Daniels's Rawlsian account and avoids the Friedian objection to that account of including too much under our healthcare rights.

A right to medical care on this basis would belong to human beings simply as such, regardless of any other fact about them as individuals (e.g. their ethnicity, their gender, their social class, their financial position, etc.). We can now return to 'solidaristic' systems of medical provision, like the NHS and similar systems in Scandinavia and elsewhere. It can be argued that such systems defend a right to medical care defined in this way better than market systems. We shall begin by considering the ideal type of a pure market in medical care. (It is doubtful whether such a pure market system exists anywhere, at least in the developed world, but that need not preclude us from asking what it *would* be like, *if* it existed. The very fact that pure markets in medical care are hard to find perhaps indicates the felt moral inappropriateness of applying unmodified market mechanisms in this case.) In an idealised pure market system for any goods, suppliers would provide the goods in question (say, medical care) to those consumers who wished for it and were able and willing to pay the price demanded by the supplier. Thus, the only sense which could be attached to the terms 'justice' and 'rights' in this context would be that every consumer has a right to, and only to, whatever goods they can afford to pay for. The system is operating 'justly' when every consumer obtains their rights in this sense, and 'unjustly' when they do not. (There might be an injustice, for example, if someone who could afford to pay for appropriate medical care was denied it on the grounds of their ethnicity, or gender, or religion, or some other irrelevant criterion.) Justice in such a system is the Rawlsian equality of opportunity. A just system is one without artificial or institutional obstacles to people's pursuing their own individual conception of the good. Of course, as in any market in any commodity, some supplier may provide the commodity without payment, out of charity, out of the pure goodness of their heart, but to provide it from charity is not to provide it as of right. Thus, in a pure market system of medical provision, medical care could not be provided as a universal human right, since entitlement to receive it would depend, not on being human and in need, but on one's ability to pay for it.

In the modern world there are purely pragmatic, non-moral factors which confuse the market situation. As health economists are fond of pointing out, there are three important respects in which the provision of medical care differs from most markets.

1 The need for medical care is more unpredictable than that for many other goods. None of us knows with any certainty when and how (if at all) we are

liable to fall ill or suffer injuries in the course of our life so that we need medical attention, and attention of a specific kind. The need for food, clothing, computers, refrigerators or cars is, by contrast, relatively predictable.

2 'Consumers', by and large, lack the relevant expertise to make unaided rational choices of the kinds of medical care they require, and have to rely on the 'providers' (the medical practitioners) to make the choices on their behalf. Something similar to this situation does, of course, exist in other fields, such as the servicing of cars owned by those who know little about the workings of the internal combustion engine, but it is rarely found in most markets.

3 In modern medicine at least, much medical care is too expensive to be paid for from the private resources of an individual on their own, unless perhaps that individual is *extremely* wealthy.

For the first and third reasons, even privately-funded medical care now tends to mean medical care funded by private *insurance*, in which individuals contribute to a common pool what they can afford, in the hope that sufficient will be available in the pool to meet any medical needs which they may have (which depends, of course, on some members of the pool not drawing from it, or drawing less from it than others). As in any insurance scheme, a certain gamble is involved. I contribute to the collective pool in order to protect myself against any risks that may arise for me and my family, but have to accept that this may mean that, if I am not ill, my contributions will go to pay for the medical care of others who are less lucky than me. This 'pooling of risks' is not genuine altruism, therefore, but 'enlightened self-interest'. I am primarily concerned, not with the medical needs of others, but with those of myself and my family, but recognise that, in the circumstances of modern medicine and the unpredictability of illness, I may need to accept the possibility that protecting my own needs means that my payments may contribute more to other people's medical welfare than my own. There is a market in 'private medicine', but it is a peculiar kind of market, a market in insurance rather than directly in medical care itself. And because of this, and because of the 'consumer's' ignorance of what is medically required, the insurance company ultimately decides what kinds of medical care may be funded from the pooled resources. Nevertheless, the right to medical care still belongs to the subscribers, not by virtue of being human, but by virtue of being able to pay their premiums (or have them paid for them by their employer).

As said earlier, even in fundamentally private systems, such as the one which exists in the US, some provision is made for medical care for those who cannot afford to pay for it themselves, and who, being unemployed, cannot have premiums paid for them by employers. Apart from private charity, there are subsidiary systems funded by the state to provide for at least the basic needs of some particularly vulnerable or deserving groups, such as the elderly poor or veterans. But these systems are so subordinate that they do not really involve recognition of a universal human right to medical provision. At most, they recognise that *some* provision must be made, as a kind of limited state charity, for the basic medical needs of disadvantaged groups. Hence, attempts to extend the system of state provision, to change the whole system to make it more like the NHS, tend to be regarded as proposals for radical change of a 'socialistic' or anti-market kind.

In a solidaristic system like the NHS, however, the situation is reversed. State provision is the core element, and privately-funded treatment (or private insurance) is regarded as peripheral and somewhat inconsistent with the basic ideology. The right to medical care, in such a non-market system, belongs to all human beings (or to citizens by virtue of being human), rather than to those who are able to pay for it. The right of everyone to medical care can be satisfied because those who are better off in society are seen as having a duty to provide the means to care for those who are most vulnerable, not just for their minimal basic needs, but for all the requirements of their vulnerability. This is not to deny that other motivations for establishing a scheme of national health insurance exist and are important – for example, the need to ensure a healthy workforce and the need referred to by Beveridge to reduce poverty by enabling all citizens as far as possible to pursue paid employment. It is only to say that the question of a *moral right* to free medical care depends above all on the vulnerability of human dignity in the face of ill health. And the medical care to which everyone is entitled is not only that which will create 'equality of opportunity', but that which will meet the medical needs of everyone, in terms of freedom from unnecessary pain, freedom from premature death, and freedom from disability, as far as these are attainable by medical means. This applies of course to *all* vulnerable and non-contributing groups, including children and disabled people. However, here we are particularly considering medical care for retired people who have, by definition, ceased to be part of the national workforce, but are still regarded as having rights to medical care, whatever their past or present contributions to funding the system may be.

The introduction of the notion of 'solidarity' into the discussion enables us to place the question of a perceived impending crisis of ageing in a new light. In a market-based system, no particular crisis seems to be created by an ageing population, though there may be some practical difficulties. Those who want medical provision in old age will still have to pay for it, and they can do this either by increasing their contributions earlier in life or by continuing, if they can afford to do so, their contributions in old age. Those who cannot afford to provide for themselves by these means can perhaps be covered by private charity or by state-funded medical care of a minimal kind, but they have no 'right', in terms of the system, to such cover. In a solidaristic system, however, the duty on the better off to provide for medical care, even for non-taxpayers, surely includes a duty to provide for those past retirement age, whether or not they pay tax, and whether or not any taxes they do pay are sufficient to cover their requirements for medical care. It is sometimes said, especially by older people themselves, that they have paid taxes all their working lives and therefore are entitled to full NHS care in their old age on the basis of *their own* past contributions. But this, though understandable, misrepresents the moral situation. Their contributions during working life were not insurance against their own old age, but part of the duty of solidarity which they themselves then had towards their fellow citizens, including those who were retired at that time. Given the loss of the value of money through inflation, especially in the costs of medical care, their past contributions almost certainly *could* not cover the full costs of care in old age. What they *have* contributed to throughout their life is the maintenance of the solidaristic system as a whole, which gives them a legitimate expectation that they should benefit from it when they cease to be taxpayers in retirement, but that is a different matter.

The ageing of the population creates a crisis for a solidaristic system like the NHS because it reduces the number of those contributing (mainly those who are younger, of working age) and increases the number of those benefiting without contributing (those who are retired from paid employment), and furthermore may be thought to be liable to increase the costs of medical care which have to be met by the contributors, if it is true that medical care for the old and frail is more expensive than that for the young and healthy. There is thus, it is suggested, a strain imposed on solidarity, as the younger contributors find their burdens in providing for others increased. We may recall the quotation from Nicholas Mays's article referred to earlier:

> It is argued that 'solidaristic', or universal, collective systems will face increasing challenges to their sustainability as rising demand for healthcare collides with the growing reluctance of the more affluent sections of the population to pay for services that will be mainly consumed by people other than themselves (Mays, 2000, p. 122).

In contrast, Houtepen and Ter Meulen (2000a and b), in reviewing the influences on solidarity in Europe, concluded that:

- The concept of solidarity can be compatible with the processes of individualisation. Indeed if individualisation is a shared and explicit value it requires the solidarity of institutions to uphold it. This can include 'market arrangements and private responsibilities' as long as this is recognised by all as a shared way to relate to each other (p. 336).
- This, however, requires a *shared* (our italics) approach by government and citizens to creating the necessary arrangements for active participation that accommodate diversity and change (p. 337). Communitarianism and similar value systems cannot meet the challenge of a pluralistic society with multiple goals and values because they are too non-specific, but 'Third Way' politics does reflect this approach.
- In essence, solidarity requires the specification of roles, whereas principles such as justice do not. They note the term 'reflective solidarity' (Dean, 1995) to describe the combination of solidarity with a 'positive approach to differences' (p. 368).

On this basis, they offer a working definition of solidarity:

> The inter-subjective experience and common action required to uphold a system of social relationships and values that complied with common standards of decency (p. 336).

Nonetheless there is a sense of 'growing reluctance' in the UK which, it might be argued, is not simply a sociological or psychological fact about the affluent – an increase in selfish concern for themselves and their families. Some might say that it rests on a legitimate sense of moral injustice. If older people have rights to medical care, the argument might go, younger, working people also have some rights to use their own income to provide for the interests and needs of themselves and their families. This too is an aspect of human dignity. As long as older people and their special medical needs remain a relatively small part of the total population, the rights of old and young can be fairly easily balanced, but the projected demographic changes will, it can be argued, undermine that equilibrium, and impose too great a burden on the young who pay the bulk of the taxation.

The ethical crisis, it would then be concluded, would arise from the need to try to combine the demands of solidarity with the old, that is, of meeting the just claims of older people, with those of justice for the young. It would be a crisis, in short, of 'intergenerational justice'.

What we need to do in the rest of this work, therefore, is, first, to examine whether this argument is valid – does the ageing of the population raise questions about justice between the generations in a system such as the NHS? We shall do this in the next chapter, by presenting and critically analysing Norman Daniels's views on the question. Daniels, as we shall see, argues that the problem of caring for older people is misconstrued if it is seen as a problem of intergenerational justice. His presentation of this view raises a number of relevant issues for our present discussion, but we shall argue that his claims, while they may apply to a system based on private insurance, do not apply to tax-funded systems like the NHS because of their different moral basis. In the latter kind of system, we argue, the problem of justice between generations can still arise. We shall then proceed, in later chapters, to further consideration of the issue of 'intergenerational justice' in systems like the NHS. The question of so-called 'rationing' or prioritisation of medical care will be analysed. We shall ask whether any system of rationing of medical care is morally justifiable, and in particular whether age in years could be a morally acceptable criterion for prioritisation, or would on the contrary constitute an intolerable 'ageism'. If it was morally acceptable, would age-based rationing resolve the question of intergenerational justice?

This will require us to consider what method of allocating medical provision can properly be described as 'rationing', and what principles of rationing (if any) can be called 'fair'. We shall argue that a fair system of rationing based on age can exist only if it can be shown that there are some relevant characteristics of different age groups as such which morally justify attributing to them different rights to medical care. Finally, we shall present and critically examine the views of the distinguished American bioethicist Dan Callahan to the effect that modern medicine has gone astray in large part through denying the significance of ageing in relation to medical needs, and in so doing has created an unnecessary crisis for itself. Callahan's views have played a particularly important part in the whole recent philosophical discussion of the problem of an ageing population, and have generated a considerable literature, at least among philosophers. They thus provide an appropriate focus for our own examination of these issues. We shall ultimately reject Callahan's position, and in Chapter 9 shall examine what remains of the idea of a crisis of ageing in the light of this.

Chapter 5

Daniels and the 'Prudential Lifespan Account'

Introduction

In the previous chapter it was argued that, if there is to be an ethical crisis of ageing in the NHS, it will be because the increasing proportions of retired people in the population will create a problem of 'intergenerational justice'. But it has been suggested that it is misleading to think of the issues concerning medical provision for an ageing population in terms of intergenerational justice. This phrase, the argument is, has strictly no meaning, so that there cannot really be any such problem, for the NHS or any other system. In this chapter, we shall consider this suggestion. It comes from the same Norman Daniels whose general position on justice in medical care was examined in Chapter 3. Once again, our procedure will be first to try to set out Daniels's position as fairly as we can, without critical comment, and only then to subject it to critical analysis. Much of what Daniels has to say about the special problems of caring for older people presupposes the general position about medical provision which has already been outlined. Where this is so, we shall avoid unnecessary repetition of points already made.

Is the problem one of 'intergenerational justice'?

Daniels's most extended account of his views about caring for older people is contained in his book *Am I My Parents' Keeper?* (Daniels, 1988), but this is a development of views expressed more briefly in a chapter of the same title (Chapter 5) in his book *Just Health Care* (Daniels, 1985), the work discussed in our own previous chapter. In *Just Health Care*, it will be remembered, Daniels argued that the right to healthcare was founded in the principle of equality of opportunity which is a key element in a Rawlsian account of justice. The most fundamental question which he needs to answer in the present context, therefore, is whether such an account of rights to medical care is not *necessarily* age-biased. He points out that 'In the US system, people over the age of 65 use health-care services at roughly 3.5 times the rate (in dollars) of those below that age' (Daniels, 1985, p. 86). Some people would argue on that basis, he goes on, that such disproportionate spending on the medical care of the older age group could not be justified on a fair equality of opportunity account, since the over-65s have already utilised all the opportunities they may have had, especially their opportunities to enter careers. Thus, it is concluded that such an account inevitably discriminates against older people: to base the right to medical care on its capacity to enable individuals to realise their opportunities, and on this alone, inevitably discrimi-nates in favour of those who still have opportunities to realise, that is, younger people. But it would be equally possible, Daniels suggests, to argue that current practice discriminates *against* the young, since expenditure on efforts to extend life marginally or to prolong dying for the older age group necessarily impacts on the young, in a realistic context of limited resources, by diverting funds which could be better spent on preventing death and alleviating suffering in children and young people.

Both arguments, in Daniels's opinion, are anyway much too crude, since they both depend on an unanalysed conception of age bias. The picture in both cases is of separate sets of people competing with one another for scarce resources. Given this picture, it then seems that we can satisfy the legitimate needs of one set (younger people) only by undermining essential values of respect for the old (the other set). We seem, in this way of thinking, to be forced to ask such questions as *how much* we owe to older people as a reward for their past services. This picture is confused, in Daniels's opinion, and this is in many ways his most original and provocative contribution to the debate about the 'crisis of ageing'. 'What makes the age problem distinctive', he says, 'is that people born at the same time (birth cohorts) age, and they are transformed successively into different age groups' (Daniels, 1985, p. 88). Different age groups, he argues, should not be regarded as different sets of people, like different social classes or genders or ethnic groups; rather, they are the same people at different stages of their lives.

The confusion arises, he says, through failing to distinguish different concepts, those of an *age group*, of a *birth cohort*, and of a *generation*. An age group consists of all those people who fall within a certain age range at a certain time (how that age range is defined will vary depending on the context). Thus, one might say that all those who have presently, in the first decade of the twenty-first century, passed their 65th birthday, but have not yet reached their 80th (say), constitute a particular age group (the 65–80-year-olds). The composition of that age group will be constantly changing, as new individuals reach the age of 65 and others pass their 80th birthday (or, of course, die). This is clearly a different concept from that of a birth cohort, which refers to a group of people born between certain dates (again, the choice of dates will depend on the context). Thus, all those born between 1 January 1930 and 31 December 1940 belong to the same birth cohort. An individual belongs to the same birth cohort throughout her life, but changes her age group as the years go by: to put it differently, birth cohorts age, but age groups don't. For instance, those born between 1930 and 1940 (provided they survived long enough) were first in the 'infancy' age group, then in the 'child-hood' group, then in the 'adolescent', and so on.

Much of the possibility of confusion of which Daniels speaks comes from the ambiguity of the third concept, that of a 'generation'. This term can be used either to refer to an age group or to a birth cohort. Thus, we may speak of the 'pre-war generation', i.e. the birth cohort of those born before the Second World War, or, equally correctly, of the 'older generation', i.e. the age group which at some particular time has passed middle age. Again, the composition of a generation in the former sense remains fixed, while that of a generation in the second sense is variable. It is because of this ambiguity that Daniels objects to the term 'intergenerational justice'. It blurs the distinction in a thoroughly misleading way between birth cohorts and age groups. It may make sense to talk about justice between the 'pre-war' and the 'post-war' generation, for example, since here we are dealing with maintaining equality between different groups of people. But it does not make sense, at least in the same way, Daniels maintains, to talk of justice between 'the older' and 'the younger' generation, since the older generation are the same people as those who were once young, as the passengers who get off the plane at Aberdeen are the same people as those who earlier boarded it at Heathrow. (The comparison just made is not, of course, made by Daniels.)

Issues of justice still arise, but it is misleading to talk of 'intergenerational' justice, since that assimilates the issues to those of justice as between different ethnic groups or genders. The problem of justice in the latter cases is that of avoiding setting up our system of resource allocation in such a way that it unfairly discriminates in favour of one group or against another. We wish, for example, to avoid systematic disadvantaging of 'black' people as opposed to 'white', and equally may wish to make sure that those born before the Second World War, who experienced harsher living conditions when they were growing up, are not disadvantaged by the system of provisions by comparison with those born later, in more prosperous times. But talk of an ethical 'crisis of ageing' within the system of medical provision implies that all those who enter the 'older age group', no matter in what circumstances they may have grown up, may be systematically disadvantaged (or advantaged) in comparison with those who happen at some time to belong to the 'younger age group'. But this, if Daniels's argument is right, would make as little sense as talk of ensuring that we do not discriminate against (or in favour of) those who disembark at Aberdeen by comparison with those who embark at Heathrow. No one is *intrinsically* young, middle-aged or old: these are different stages in the same person's life.

Hence, the problem of justice for 'the old', whether in relation to medical care or to anything else, cannot be thought of as that of ensuring a fair distribution of resources between two separate groups of people. Rather, we have to think of it against the background, or, as Daniels puts it, in the frame, of a general theory of distributive justice, as a particular corollary which follows from the fact that human beings age, i.e. that human lives and needs change over time. Distributive justice in general requires that all human beings should be treated equally, except when there is some relevant reason for discrimination. To take a crude example, there are good reasons for providing obstetric services for women but not for men; but there are no good reasons for providing better obstetric services for white women than for black women. But given that each individual's life changes over time, equal treatment for men and women, or for black and white people, means that all parts of each individual's life should be fairly considered. This does not, however, necessarily mean that the needs of each phase are the same or equal. Fairness means rather that the differing needs of each phase of life must be fairly met, whether it is a male life or a female life, a white or a black person's life. The 'moral relevance' of age in distributive contexts, Daniels proposes, lies in the fact that 'considering age can produce an allocation that makes the life of *each person better off* . . . as a whole' (Daniels, 1988, p. 92: Daniels's italics).

On this view, then, the problem of distributive justice in relation to age groups is one of deciding what are legitimate 'transfers' between different phases of the same individual's life. The question to be asked, in the terms of his own theory of medical justice, is this: what distribution of medical care resources between childhood, working life and old age would best enable each individual to enjoy the normal opportunity range, or more generally would make every individual's life equally good as a whole? The implication of Daniels's way of expressing this is that, in addition to the general concept of a 'normal opportunity range', there is, or may be, what might be called an 'age-relative normal opportunity range' (*see* Daniels, 1988, p. 74), that is, a differentiation in the normal opportunity range based on the needs and capacities of the age group under consideration. The normal opportunity range for children, for people in their prime, and for those of retirement age and older would differ, so that to ensure 'equality of opportunity' for everyone would mean to ensure that all were able equally to enjoy the *appropriate* opportunities for each phase of life through which they passed. This would be what a 'prudent' person would choose for themselves if setting up a system behind a 'veil of ignorance'.

This is the basis of what Daniels calls the 'Prudential Lifespan Account'. On this account, a fair distribution of medical resources between different age groups would be that which a prudent rational deliberator would embody in institutions under which she is prepared to live her own life in all its phases. Such a prudent deliberator might be prepared, for instance, to 'save' some resources that might otherwise be used in childhood, or in young adulthood, in order to be able to meet needs which might arise later in life. This is the same kind of prudence which leads us to save from our income during working life (thereby denying ourselves some more immediate satisfactions) in order to provide a pension for ourselves after retirement. The aim of the saving in both cases is to ensure the best possible life as a whole, or 'lifespan'. In order to be able to do this, deliberators would need to be able to abstract from the point of view of the particular phase of life which they currently occupied – to set aside, for these purposes, the concerns of youth as such in order to look at their life from a point of view which was not that of any particular age because it considered their life as a whole. This would be a kind of assumed ignorance of their actual age at the time of deliberation. In particular, they would need, Daniels argues, to set aside their current age-related life plan. A young person's life plan, for instance, is liable to focus on such things as the need to find a satisfactory career, whereas in middle or old age that is not so likely to be central to our plans for the rest of our life. What young deliberators would need to do would be to think what they would be likely to regard as important when they are older, and to consider the relative importance of their present concerns in contributing to the overall desirability of their life as a whole. The feat of abstraction that this would require can be compared in some ways to Rawls's notion of a 'veil of ignorance', though Daniels denies that it is strictly the same, because the justification for the assumed restrictions on knowledge is different. 'The restriction on knowledge of one's own age', he says, 'is a way of keeping our prudent choice problem within the frame that excludes transfers across the boundaries between persons' (Daniels, 1988, p. 67). That is, it has to do with transfers between different stages of the same person's life, rather than, as with Rawls's device, on fair distribution between different persons. Rawls's device is, as Daniels says, 'an attempt to model an underlying ideal of the nature of moral agents' (id., ibid.), as beings who think in an *impersonal* way, considering what would be in the interest of *any* person, rather than specifically what is in *their own* self-interest. Daniels's concern is rather with what is in *one's own* long-term, as opposed to short-term, self-interest.

As already stated, the idea of 'saving' resources, as a prudent means of making one's life as a whole better, is already familiar to us from such contexts as provision for pensions. Daniels would also say that the same basic principle applies, though with a twist, when pensions are based on the taxation of those who are still working. The twist is that *my* pension is paid for by *others'* sacrifice; but, he would say, the principle remains the same in that, in so doing, the taxpayers are also providing for their own future pensions by making themselves eligible to benefit in their turn when they leave full-time paid employment. Daniels then attempts to apply this to the medical care situation, both in the US and in the NHS. (We must remember that we are simply reporting Daniels's views at this point without criticism: our own view differs sharply from his, as will be seen later.) One essential function of the NHS, as Daniels sees things, is that of saving in this sense. Employed workers, through their taxes, pay the great bulk of the costs of the medical care system as a whole, way beyond what is required to meet their own present medical needs, in order to pay for the care of children (who have not yet started employment) and those who have retired from paid work (cf. Daniels, 1988, p. 44). The special feature of the present situation, which he thinks prudent deliberators must take into account, is that the increase in the post-retirement lifespan requires a greater rate of savings:

> If lifetime earnings are held constant, but lifespan is extended, then the rate at which resources must be transferred from early stages of life to later stages must be increased. We must take more from our young and middle ages to finance our later ones (Daniels, 1988, pp. 77f).

This account, he goes on to argue, would allow in certain circumstances for something which could be regarded as a form of age-based rationing of medical care. A prudent person making a judgement about the distribution of medical care resources over her entire life might, for example, prefer a scheme in which greater resource was used in enabling her to reach a normal lifespan to one which saved resources in that respect in order to enable her to live a longer than normal time *if* she was fortunate enough to reach a normal lifespan. Putting the same point in more concrete terms, such a deliberator might think it better to spend money on medical care and surgery in her younger years which would give her a good chance of reaching the age of, say, 75 than to save resources on such care in order to have more available, if she reached 75 anyway, to provide the kinds of treatment she would need to gain further years of life thereafter.

On page 87 of his *Am I My Parents' Keeper* (Daniels, 1988), Daniels outlines two possible alternative schemes of distribution by way of illustration. The first, which he calls Scheme A, could be described as a form of age-based rationing. Under this scheme, 'No one over age 70 or 75 . . . is eligible to receive any of several high-cost, life-extending technologies such as dialysis, transplant surgery, or extensive by-pass surgery'. This would release resources for developing these technologies to benefit younger people, thus enabling more younger people to reach the age of 70 or 75. The second scheme, which he calls Scheme L (for lottery), would reject anything that could be seen as age-based rationing and allocates according to medical need, regardless of the age of patients. Given the greater medical needs of older people, this in effect involves making fewer resources available for the care of younger patients in order to ensure that the needs of older people can be provided for. The consequence of it would therefore be that fewer young people would survive to 70 or 75, but that more old people would survive beyond that age. Daniels expresses this difference in terms of probabilities, taking an extreme scenario in order to make the point clearer. 'Scheme A might offer a 1.0 probability of reaching age 75 (and dying right away), and Scheme L might give a 0.5 probability of reaching 50 and a 0.5 probability of reaching 100' (Daniels, 1988, p. 87).

Scheme A could properly be seen as a form of age-based rationing, since it involves prioritising the life-preserving care of younger people over extending the lives of older people. Those who do manage to survive beyond 75 will, under this plan, be denied access to medical care which might prolong their lives further. Is this objectionably discriminating? Daniels would argue that it is not, since it does not discriminate in favour of one *group* of people (the young) as against another, quite separate, group (the old), but is what would in his opinion be preferred by *any* prudent deliberator as a way of distributing resources across the lifespan so as to make her own life as a whole better. In this sense, it treats all people equally, and so justly. 'An institution that treats the young and the old differently', he contends, 'will, over time, still treat people equally' (Daniels, 1988, p. 41). People's medical needs change at different stages in their lives, and it is only prudent for each of us, in choosing the system of distribution of medical care resources, to allow for this variation. He concludes, therefore, that 'we cannot claim that age-rationing is always unjust' (Daniels, 1988, p. 89). It does not follow from this, of course (and Daniels does not think it follows), that *any* form of age-based rationing is morally justifiable. What is crucial is whether the allocation is such that a prudent deliberator would choose it for herself as a way of making her life as a whole better. If the reason for denying older people certain forms of care were, for example, simply a desire to contain the overall costs of the system, where a prudent deliberator would choose those forms of care in old age, then the scheme could not be justified by Daniels's argument.

A particular case which Daniels discusses in more detail is that of long-term care for older people. Under this heading he includes not only medical and mental healthcare, but also nursing care, rehabilitative therapy, personal care services and social services. The need for such care, as he says, increases with age, so that the ageing of society as a whole necessarily makes it urgent to consider the provision of long-term care. Daniels has forceful criticisms of the US system for its neglect of long-term care, especially the non-medicalised aspects of it. The non-medical elements of long-term care, he argues, have exactly the same moral purpose as the medical, namely, 'to maintain or restore or compensate for the losses of normal functioning' (Daniels, 1988, p. 106). In particular, they maintain, restore or compensate for the loss of the individual's *independence*, a crucial element in an individual's opportunity to carry out otherwise reasonable parts of a plan of life. In this sense, having one's house cleaned or one's shopping done, or having a place to meet others socially, may be at least as important to an old person's wellbeing, and so as much of a right, as access to high-technology medical care. (One can agree with this point in general without accepting Daniels's rather contrived attempt to relate it to 'opportunity': long-term care contributes to a person's wellbeing in the sense of preserving her sense of self-respect, whether or not it enables her to carry out her life plan.) Daniels is therefore willing to argue that rationing of acute medical services to pay for better long-term care in old age is justifiable in terms of the Prudential Lifespan

Account. He has some favourable comments on the NHS from this point of view, saying:

> It is possible to understand some of the rationing choices made in the British National Health Service, which provides considerable home care to the partially disabled, as a choice made in this spirit (Daniels, 1988, p. 109).

Whether this is as true now as it was when Daniels was writing may be doubted, especially in view of the debate about the proposals made in the Report of the Royal Commission chaired by Sir Stewart Sutherland (Sutherland, 1999), rejected by the UK Government up to now, though largely implemented in Scotland by the Scottish Executive (*see* Appendix 1). More will be said about long-term care in our own conclusions.

Individual prudence and social justice

Daniels thus presents us with a distinctive way of thinking about the crisis of ageing which seems to avoid the ethical problems of 'intergenerational justice'. His differentiation between age groups, birth cohorts and generations certainly helps to avoid certain kinds of conceptual confusion into which it is otherwise easy to fall, and so aids clarity on the issues which confront us. Nevertheless, he seems to us to be open to criticism from the point of view of the NHS and similar publicly-funded systems, and does not show that we can avoid thinking of an ethical crisis of ageing in such systems. The core of his account of the ethics of medical care for older people is the idea of the 'prudent deliberator'. The fair way to allocate medical resources, and the care which they support, as between different age groups, he contends, is to do so in a way which a prudent rational deliberator would choose if she were considering what would be most likely to make her life as a whole maximally desirable. She would have to decide how much should be spent on the typical medical needs of childhood, how much on those of youth and middle age, and how much on those of old age. This is explicitly compared, as we have seen, with the way in which we decide how much of our income we should set aside when young in order to make adequate provision for our anticipated pension needs when retired. Our central criticism of this account is that, while it might make some kind of sense if we were dealing with an individual's provision for her own medical needs, it sounds much less plausible when we are concerned with a centrally financed and organised system. If each of us were faced with an array of medical insurance schemes, offering different patterns of distribution of care over the lifespan, then each of us could choose the one which best suited our own conception of what would make our lives best as a whole. But, even in the US, this is not usually the situation. People do not normally have a choice of schemes differentiated in that way, but are compelled to accept the particular scheme favoured by their employer (or sometimes, if they are lucky, between more than one scheme offered by their employer). It is certainly not the case in the NHS, where decisions about distribution of resources are made, not by individuals for their own case, but centrally, in the light of general and impersonal considerations.

Just because it is a non-market system, decisions about allocation of resources in the NHS are made centrally and impersonally. The NHS is an *institution*, not an individual or a random collection of individuals. Its decisions are therefore institutional decisions. Those who make them are not individuals, disposing of their own income according to their own preferences, but public servants disposing of public revenues according to some generally accepted standards of justice. In the particular case of distribution of medical resources between young and old, what matters from this point of view is whether it is *right* by these standards to spend more on keeping young people alive to the age of 70 than is spent on prolonging the life of older people beyond that age. This cannot be decided simply by consulting those involved at any particular time, say in an opinion poll, about what they would think prudent in their own case, both because there would almost certainly be a variety of different opinions among them on that issue, and because the decision has to apply over time and will therefore apply to many who were not there to be consulted when the opinion poll was taken. The root mistake in Daniels's position is the attempt to link justice and prudence. In his terms, prudence is a virtue of individual decisions about their own lives: it is a matter of thinking in terms of long-term rather than short-term self-interest. Justice is, as Rawls puts it, a virtue of institutions. It is concerned, not with self-interest as such, but with balancing the *rights* of different individuals in such a way as to ensure that everyone has equal rights. Choosing a scheme of medical provision which will be prudent from one's own point of view is a different sort of decision from choosing a just allocation of resources between young and old.

This leads on to a further criticism. While it is perfectly true that from some points of view it is useful to regard those who have retired as the same people as those who were at an earlier stage in their lives part of the working population, it does not follow that we have thereby dissolved or defused the problem of 'intergenerational justice'. Questions of intergenerational justice do not, of course, arise for us when we are making decisions about our own lives: if I am now young, I cannot regard my later self as another person to whom I need to be 'fair'. But decisions made in collective bodies such as the NHS do concern groups of people who, at any given time, are distinct from each other. Those who now belong to the 'older generation' are of course the same people as those who *previously* belonged to the 'younger generation'; but they are certainly not the same people as those who *now* belong to the younger generation. The resource allocation decisions that have to be made in the NHS concern distribution between those who at any given time belong to the younger and the older generations, and these are always, as just argued, distinct groups of people. There thus seems to be no reason, at least prima facie, why there should not be problems about justice between these distinct groups, as between any others, such as ethnic groups, genders, social classes and so on. The respective rights of these different groups may conflict, and justice would require this conflict to be resolved.

We can return at this point to Daniels's claim that in the NHS those of working age are 'saving' for their own old age as well as providing for their current needs. We have already touched upon this issue earlier, but it is useful in view of what has just been said to repeat our reasons for thinking this claim to be misleading. In a system such as the NHS, those in work pay their taxes, not just to provide for their own old age but also, and importantly, to pay for the needs of those who are unable to pay taxes themselves, either because they are unemployable because of disability or chronic illness, or because they are too young to have started work, or because they have retired from paid work. (It is the last-named group, of course, which mainly concerns us here.) Workers are saving for their own future, as was said in the last chapter, only in the sense that they are helping to ensure the continuance of a system which will eventually benefit them in the same way when they have ceased to work. But this is not at all the kind of saving to which Daniels refers, as part of his Prudential Lifespan Account. It is not like making contributions to a private pension scheme, but more like paying taxes to maintain a state retirement pension. The moral principle behind the NHS, as argued earlier, is that of solidarity, of the better-off members of society contributing to protect the more vulnerable members, rather than that of risk sharing, which underpins private insurance schemes. (This is not incompatible with accepting that there is an element of risk pooling in the NHS, and thus an element of prudence in our motivation for supporting it. It is simply to say that what is distinctive about systems such as the NHS from a moral point of view is the element of solidarity, and that it is this which may create issues of justice.)

Daniels's attempt to dissolve the question of intergenerational justice thus fails, because his Prudential Lifespan Account applies only to the decisions made by individuals about their own future medical needs, where no question of justice can arise, and does not apply to collective systems such as the NHS, which is where justice must be an issue. It does not follow from his failure, however, that there will be an ethical crisis of ageing, resulting from intractable problems of intergenerational justice. To draw that conclusion, it would be necessary to show both that the demands made on the medical care system by an increasing number of older people must create intolerable demands on the resources provided (mainly) by the taxes of younger people, and also that older people are morally entitled to make these demands. In order to consider these issues clearly, we shall first, in the next chapter, consider the ethical principles of rationing and prioritisation in relation to medical care.

Chapter 6

Ethics and resource allocation

The meaning of 'rationing'

If there is to be a crisis of ageing in the NHS and similar systems, we have argued, it will be an *ethical* one. The fear that lies behind the perception of an impending crisis is that the shift in the age balance of the population might make it difficult or even impossible to sustain that sense of solidarity which provides the ethical underpinning of this kind of system. In the NHS, the taxes of the whole population, including those who are healthy, provide the resources to fund the care of the unhealthy, and (more relevant to our theme) the taxes of those young enough to be in employment provide most of the resources to fund the care of those who have retired from employment (though of course retired people themselves are in many cases also liable to tax). No problem of fairness would arise if, in paying their taxes, the employed people were simply insuring themselves against future illness or disability, since that would be a question of prudent saving rather than of distributive justice. Daniels's idea, as we have seen, is that this is in fact what is the case in the NHS, but we argued in the last chapter that, while his 'Prudential Lifespan Account' might apply to the purchase of private medical insurance, in systems like the NHS we cannot avoid questions of distributive justice. Someone taking out private medical insurance for herself and/or her family is making a prudent investment for her own/her family's future. But the NHS is constituted by the state, to care for the medical needs of the whole community, in which at any given time the 'older generation' and the 'younger generation' are different sets of people, each with different rights and claims. Those claims must be balanced fairly, and the perception is that this is what becomes difficult when the older generation, with its disproportionately costly demands on the system, becomes a significantly larger section of the population than it has traditionally been.

The resources available for medical care are inevitably finite, both in the sense that *all* human resources are finite, and in the sense that the portion of total resources to be dedicated to medical care is limited by the need to cater for other public needs, such as education, housing, policing, national defence, road-building and so on. Distributive justice in relation to medical care is a matter of allocating the 'medical' portion of total resources fairly between different uses, either in the sense of the care of different conditions, or in the care for different groups in the population (in the case which most concerns us, groups defined by age). Differential allocation in either sense is what we want to call 'rationing'. This term, especially in the context of medical care, tends to raise hackles. Rationing is often seen as intrinsically unethical in such cases, and certainly politicians like to avoid using it, preferring some more innocuous-sounding word like 'prioritisation'. But all that the word means, as we use it, is the sharing out of some scarce resource among different people according to some rational principle, and that does not seem to be *intrinsically* unethical (although it could be, if the rational principle in question were not also a moral principle: rationing by price, as in a market system, for example, would not be an ethical form of rationing). 'Prioritisation' would then be simply the specific form of rationing in which the allocation attached greater weight to some things (in the medical case, to certain forms of treatment or certain categories of patients) than to others.

Rationing in this sense is not only ethically acceptable in the right circumstances, but can actually in some cases be ethically *required*. To see this, we can consider the case of food rationing in Britain during the Second World War. Because wartime conditions interfered with some of the normal sources of supply of food, the stocks of food available to provide for the British population were limited. On the other hand, it was essential, for moral as well as other reasons, to ensure that *every* member of the population was as well nourished as possible. If the normal market rules of supply and demand had been followed, those best able to afford to buy food would have been better nourished than those who were less wealthy, and that would have been unjust. A rationing scheme was therefore introduced to equalise everyone's entitlement to sufficient food to keep them reasonably well nourished. Everyone, no matter what their income, had ration 'coupons' entitling them (on cash payment) to specified quantities of different types of food. Thus, the well off could not use their greater wealth to buy more than their fair share of the food available, which left enough for the less well off to be able to get their fair share. This general equality was quite compatible with a form of 'prioritisation' which entitled some groups to greater shares, not on the basis of their income, but on the basis of their special needs. Thus, children were entitled to special provision (e.g. of orange juice) because of the need to protect their growth, as representing the future of the community as a whole; those involved in heavy manual labour, of crucial national importance, were entitled to extra rations because of the additional physical demands made on them. Thus, in this case a rationing scheme, including prioritisation in some cases, could be seen as a positive requirement of ethics.

Some would argue that this model could not be applied in the field of medical provision. The only ethically justifiable allocation of medical resources, they would say, is one based on strict equality. Every individual should get exactly the same amount, no matter what differences between them existed – no matter what their social class, or gender, or income, or ethnic identity, or (and here we come close to home) age in years. Any other distribution would necessarily, on this view, constitute unfair discrimination and so be unethical. One way in which even those who hold to this form of egalitarianism are sometimes willing to qualify it is to accept a need to prioritise the care *for some conditions* over that for others. They might be willing to say, for example, that more resource might justly be devoted to lifesaving treatment than to, say, cosmetic surgery for pure reasons of vanity. Their reason for accepting this would be that we could perhaps all agree that saving life makes more of a moral claim on us than beautifying someone's appearance. Once we get away from such obvious contrasts, of course, it might be more difficult to achieve consensus on priorities (a question we shall return to later), but the general principle that prioritisation on such grounds might be morally acceptable or even required might be granted by at least some critics of rationing. This sort of prioritisation is different from that described above in the wartime food rationing scheme, since it refers not to prioritising the needs of specific *groups of people* (manual workers, children), but to prioritising certain kinds of *treatment*, which might be needed, after all, by anyone from any background and of any age. In particular, those who oppose rationing of medical care, even when they are willing to qualify their opposition in the way just described, still normally object to prioritising the needs of the young over the old or vice versa. This is called 'ageism', and is felt by those who support this line of argument to be as much a form of unjust discrimination as sexism or racism, which everyone in a liberal society would reject as morally unjustifiable.

An example of this line of thinking can be found in the essay by John Grimley Evans already referred to in an earlier chapter. Grimley Evans declares:

> From these I conclude that in times of peace British national values include the equality of citizens in their relation to the institutions of the state and acknowledgement of, and respect for, the uniqueness of individuals regardless of their physical or mental attributes. From the last follows the equal right of all citizens to live as they wish so long as they do not impede the like rights of others. If these ideas are indeed embodied in the ideology of British society, ageism, as well as racism and sexism, will be unethical (Grimley Evans, 1997, p. 116).

This is Grimley Evans's main ethical argument against rationing of medical care, at least by age. In other words, he, like many others, equates age-based rationing with ageism, and, since he assumes ageism to be clearly unjust in the same way that sexism and racism are, he concludes (logically, given these premises) that age-based rationing is unjust. That conclusion may well be correct, but it seems to us to require much more subtle argument than this to support it, since Grimley Evans's premises are not as self-evidently true as he assumes.

First, we must question whether justice necessarily requires equal treatment of all. In what is one of the classic philosophical definitions of distributive justice, Aristotle says 'if the people involved are not equal, they will not [justly] receive equal shares; indeed, whenever equals receive unequal shares, or unequals equal shares, in a distribution, that is the source of quarrels and accusations' (Aristotle, *Nicomachean Ethics*, quoted from Solomon and Murphy, 2000, p. 40). As it is sometimes expressed more succinctly, distributive justice is a matter of treating equals equally and unequals unequally. Grimley Evans might argue that this is still compatible with his position, since he would claim that liberal (or, as he puts it, 'British national') ideology requires us to treat all citizens as equal, and so to be treated equally. But this would be confusing. Liberal ideology does indeed, as he says, require 'acknowledgement of, and respect for, the uniqueness of individuals regardless of their physical or mental attributes'. But it does not follow from that that it requires that every individual should receive an equal share of any good which is to be distributed. Indeed, it could be argued that respect for individuality requires recognition of individual differences, for example in their needs, and therefore different (if necessary, unequal) shares. This accords not only with Aristotle's definition, but also with our ordinary moral intuitions. The example of wartime rationing shows that. It would be considered by most people to be unjust that someone who did heavy manual work, and therefore had greater nutritional needs, should be given exactly the same food ration as someone who needed less, say, because they did much lighter and more sedentary work, or did no work at all. Justice, and indeed humanity, could not countenance that the latter received insufficient food to meet their smaller needs; but it would require that they did not receive the same share of available food reserves as the heavy manual worker.

In somewhat the same way, in medical care, it could not be just to use the same amount of available resources to provide for some relatively trivial need, say, treating teenage acne, as for something more serious, say, treatment to alleviate severe pain or to prevent premature death. These examples have been deliberately chosen as representing as far as possible clear instances of 'trivial' and 'serious' medical needs. Acne is, of course, a very serious problem for the person who has it, but a *just* allocation must be based on a more detached or 'objective' criterion of seriousness, and most would agree that a life-threatening illness is, in that objective sense, a more serious problem than the travails of adolescence. In other cases, as said already, it is, of course, much harder to rank medical needs on this scale, and that problem will need to be addressed shortly. But, for the moment, the examples at least show that not all medical needs are equal, or deserve equal resources, in a system based on justice. Justice does not require strict, mathematical equality of treatment; but what it does require is that deviations from strict equality need to be justified by being shown to arise from *morally relevant* differences between people, as the greater needs of heavy manual workers were seen as morally relevant to giving them a greater share of the available food. This is the reason why such things as sexism and racism are morally objectionable. Differences of sex do of course *in some respects* require differences in medical treatment. Men, for example, do not need treatment for the complications of pregnancy and women do not require treatment for testicular cancer. But there are many respects in which the medical needs of men and women do not differ at all, and there are no respects in which the medical needs of one sex are as such deserving of *unequal* attention. Similar points may be made about differences in ethnicity, or so-called 'race': there is nothing about a difference in skin colour or cultural background which could conceivably be seen by a rational person as justifying inequalities of medical treatment.

The question that we need to address in this work is whether age in years is a morally relevant criterion for awarding unequal shares, or whether ageism is, as Grimley Evans implies, as morally objectionable as racism or sexism. (Ageism could consist, of course, *either* in attending more to the medical needs of the young than of the old *or* the reverse). If we go back to our account of a possible crisis of ageing for the NHS, would it be unfair to expect younger taxpayers to shoulder the burden of increased medical costs created by a much greater elderly population, and thus to divert resources from their own needs and those of their children and other dependants? Or would it be unfair to deny provision for, or give a lower priority to, the medical needs of older people in order to reduce the burden on the younger generation? There would be no crisis if it could be shown that neither sort of unfairness would arise in the projected situation. This could be shown in one of two, very different, ways. First, it might be argued that the genuine medical *needs* (as opposed to the factual *demands* on the medical services) of older people, just because they are older, are intrinsically less than those of younger, so that satisfying the *rights* of older people to medical care, when those rights are properly understood, does not create an intolerable burden on the system and those who provide its resources. This is, in effect, the position of Daniel Callahan, to be considered in the next chapter. Alternatively, it could be contended that it is wrong to categorise medical needs by age, just as it would be to classify them by sex or ethnicity. As in the latter cases, there are, of course, types of medical need which tend to be characteristic of old age (or of youth), but, first, these needs are not entirely confined to the age group in question, and secondly, it could be argued that there is no moral relevance to their association with particular phases of life. If so, then no question of unfairness to the young, and so no 'ethical crisis', would arise in the envisaged situation, even though there would undoubtedly be practical problems of a political nature, and other types of ethical problem. There would then be no basis for advocating any form of *age-based* rationing as a solution to the crisis. This will be our own final position, arrived at partly by our critique of Callahan, and will be explained more fully in the final chapter.

Needs and justice in the NHS

It has already been admitted in this chapter that, while some evaluations of medical needs as relatively 'trivial' or 'serious' are fairly easy to make and would be generally agreed, in most cases such evaluations are much more difficult and contentious. In a pure market system, which effectively rations medical care by price, this problem can be solved with relative ease. Consumer preferences will decide, as in any market, how resources are allocated. The preferences of different groups of consumers may, of course, conflict, but in a market the preferences of those who carry the most clout (who have the most spending power) will prevail. But in a system based on the principle of solidarity, the problem is more complicated. Allocations must be just, that is, must be determined by what is morally right, rather than by what most people happen to want. At the same time, since collective funds are being allocated, decisions about allocation must be made by some central body that will be accountable, in a democratic society, to the elected representatives of the citizens who are benefiting from the scheme. This body will therefore have to make its allocations in a socially responsible way, balancing the claims of one group against another in a way that is explicit and can be generally accepted. Daniels and Sabin (1997) distinguish two problems here, which they call the problem of 'legitimacy' and the problem of 'fairness'. In this paper, they are thinking mainly about problems facing US managed care organisations (MCOs) or health maintenance organisations (HMOs) rather than about public systems like the NHS, but they acknowledge in a later paper, written for a British publication (Sabin and Daniels, 2002) that similar problems of legitimacy and fairness arise in both situations. As has been said in an earlier chapter, the US system, though founded on 'the value of individual responsibility and a strong national preference for addressing problems through markets rather than government' (Sabin and Daniels, 2002, p. 141), is not a pure market system, and the introduction of important elements of centralised control in the form of MCOs and HMOs is one way in which it has deviated from a pure market.

In the 1997 paper, these authors describe the legitimacy problem as follows:

> Why or when should a patient or clinician who thinks an uncovered service is appropriate or even 'medically necessary' accept as legitimate the limit-setting decisions of a MCO? (Daniels and Sabin, 1997, p. 304).

It is concerned with the *authority* of the organisation in question to make such moral decisions. The fairness problem, on the other hand, is stated as:

> When does a patient or clinician who thinks an uncovered service appropriate or even medically necessary have sufficient reason to accept as fair the limit-setting decisions of a managed care organization? (Daniels and Sabin, 1997, p. 305).

In the later paper, these authors say that:

> Legitimacy refers to the conditions under which moral authority over resource allocation decisions should be placed in the hands of private organisations (e.g. US health plans) or public agencies (e.g. UK health authorities). Fairness refers to the conditions under which patients, clinicians and the public have sufficient reason to accept a disappointing public or private resource allocation decision as fair (Sabin and Daniels, 2002, p. 142).

These two issues, they go on to say, are distinct. It is perfectly possible, for instance, according to them, for a legitimate authority to make unfair decisions.

Both legitimacy and fairness are required, however, for acceptable allocation decisions in medical care in any system that is not, or not entirely, determined by market forces. Because the decisions must be made by moral criteria, the body which makes the decisions must have moral authority. Its allocation policies must be 'reasonable' in reconciling the needs of individuals with those of the group covered as a whole. But this is not enough: 'the rationales for these policies must also be "transparent" or readily available to all of the concerned stakeholders' (Sabin and Daniels, 2002, p. 142). And the policies must be open to revision over time, and therefore 'subject to appeal' (id., ibid.). In other words, its decisions must not only be fair by its own standards, but must be seen to be fair by those affected by them.

This is where the difficulties in rationing for publicly-funded and managed organisations arise. As Sabin and Daniels point out, the UK and the US (indeed, one might say all modern societies) are pluralistic societies with no universally accepted values which could be used in making decisions about rationing and prioritisation. The problem for the NHS is more severe than for the US MCOs, for two reasons: first, that its coverage is meant to include *all citizens* rather than a particular group who choose to be covered, so that the potential diversity of values among 'stakeholders' is all the greater; and secondly, as Sabin and Daniels themselves recognise (op. cit., p. 145), that 'the NHS is expected to provide any treatment that is truly beneficial'. But both the NHS and the HMOs (fairly or not) are often criticised on the grounds that their allocation decisions are made for purely *economic* reasons (to cut costs) rather than on a basis of justice. Representatives of special interest groups, whether bodies representing sufferers from particular conditions or practitioners of particular medical specialties (or both), claim that to deny particular types of treatment to those patients that they represent, or to give their condition a lower priority for resources than others, is 'unfair'. In the absence of shared criteria for deciding what way of sharing resources between different groups of patients is just, there seems no way to resolve such arguments. But they must be resolved if a structure like the NHS is to be seen as morally, as well as legally, 'legitimate' and if the sense of social solidarity is to be maintained in the face of necessarily limited resources.

Both the articles by Sabin and Daniels referred to are primarily attempts to show how the problem of legitimacy can be resolved for MCOs in the US. But in the earlier article they claim that the legitimacy and fairness problems facing these US private institutions 'have their analogues in public systems such as the British National Health Service in Great Britain or the Canadian systems' (Daniels and Sabin, 1997, p. 348). And in the later article they suggest that the NHS can learn from the experience of some health organisations in the US 'struggling to achieve legitimacy and to set limits fairly in an unjust health care system' (Sabin and Daniels, 2002, p. 155). They refer explicitly in the earlier article to the national commissions established in recent years by the Dutch, Norwegian. Danish and Swedish governments in an attempt to articulate general principles to govern prioritisation in medical care (the Swedish report has been cited already in the present work). While not rejecting such attempts to get agreement on general principles, however, they see the main problem as that of establishing the legitimacy of *specific* decisions, such as denial of a transplant to a particular patient. Their solution to the latter problem, which they illustrate by examples from US MCOs, is essentially procedural: it consists in establishing the legitimacy of a decision-making body by making that body *accountable* to the public, in the sense of making the reasons for that particular decision available for general public discussion:

> In circumstances like this, where values conflict, accountability for reasonableness calls for resolution through a deliberative process. It specifies that the process should be accessible to the public, draw on relevant reasons (the needs of individuals and of the population), make its rationales as well as its conclusions widely available, and seek to improve its practices and policies over time by responding to appeals, calls for revision, and other opportunities for learning (Sabin and Daniels, 2002, p. 143).

Their point can be illustrated by one of the examples they consider, the decision about whether to cover Viagra considered by an HMO called Harvard Pilgrim Health Care in 1998. The question to be considered was:

> Should Viagra be regarded as a 'treatment' to be covered like medications for asthma, diabetes or migraines, or should it be seen as an 'enhancement' or 'lifestyle' drug and not be covered at all, in the same way that cosmetic surgery is not covered? (Sabin and Daniels, 2002, p. 144).

The HMO had an Ethics Advisory Group, whose function was to offer non-binding advice about the ethical aspects of such questions, and which was crucially involved in the debate on Viagra. Its discussion at first tended to favour the view that Viagra was a mere enhancement drug, until one woman member interjected that sex was not an optional matter of 'lifestyle', but was now recognised as 'an essential aspect of our being' (id., ibid.). Her interjection changed the course of the debate, and the group eventually advised the HMO that Viagra should not be regarded as a 'mere enhancement' but that nevertheless, because of the cost considerations, 'the value of adding coverage for Viagra had to be compared to the value provided by alternative uses of the funds' (Sabin and Daniels, 2002, p. 145). That is, there could be no guarantee that there would be funds available to cover Viagra if other drugs provided better value. The cost factor, the group concluded, ought to be frankly acknowledged by the organisation. Sabin and Daniels accept that such acknowledgement of the relevance of costs to decisions of this kind would be harder in the NHS, since, as they say in the passage already quoted, it is expected to provide any truly beneficial treatment. (In fact, in the initial UK discussion about Viagra, the cost factor was acknowledged, but its significance was diminished by treating the drug as a mere enhancement in most cases, and so not to be prescribed on the NHS except in those few instances where a case for genuine medical benefit – or medical reason for loss of potency – could be established.)

There are several elements in this example that are relevant to our discussion. First, the example makes it clear that real debate about rationing begins only when it is agreed that some treatment is medically beneficial (rather than simply an 'enhancement'). The debate concerns the relative priority of different treatments, *all* of which are in their own way medically beneficial, but which have to compete for a share of limited resources. Secondly, Sabin and Daniels are making a point about the need for transparency in rationing decisions if legitimacy in their sense is to be secured. This seems an obviously valid point. One common criticism of the rationing decisions which do inevitably take place in the NHS has been that they are seldom, if ever, made explicit. Proper public consultation about rationing decisions would make the cost constraints on providing medical services more widely known, and thus make it clear, and why, that not everything which was beneficial could be provided, or at least given the same priority for provision. But it does not seem, even from considering this example, that they are right to treat the solution to the fairness and legitimacy problems as *purely* procedural. In order to establish legitimacy, the *reasons* for the rationing decision also have to be made available to the public, and (especially in the case of a system like the NHS which is universal and is funded out of general taxation) have to be open to public debate and questioning. This leads on to a third point. Although the example given concerns a decision about the availability of a particular medication, the reasons given for and against coverage are *general* in character. They depend on general views about the place of sexual activity in our lives – is it just something which may 'enhance' them, in the way in which, say, a face-lift to make one feel better might, or is it something 'essential' to healthy relationships between couples? In other words, Sabin and Daniels play down too much the importance of consideration of general principles of prioritisation. If the public are to be convinced about the desirability or otherwise of providing (in this case) Viagra on the NHS, the arguments of general principle on the two sides will have to be presented to them. This implies in turn that it is possible to appeal to at least some shared general principles which can provide a basis for rational argument. Despite the pluralism of Western liberal societies referred to earlier, the resort to rational argument implies that common values can be *established*, even if they are not immediately evident before the debate begins.

The fourth, and in some ways most important, point which emerges is that the debate about the acceptability of rationing by age is different in character from the debate about rationing particular drugs or other forms of treatment. It is what might be called a 'second-order' debate, concerning the relevance of a particular sort of reason for making 'first-order' decisions about the rationing of particular treatments. Just as, in the Viagra example cited above, the discussion about the rationing of this particular drug involved a general, and almost 'philosophical', examination of the place of sex in human life, so numerous individual rationing decisions may require us to consider our attitudes to old age, and its place in the general pattern of human life. But there will also be a difference from the Viagra case. That concerned a particular type of treatment for a particular condition, and the question to be decided was whether, or to what extent, that treatment counted as medically beneficial. If (as was agreed in this case) it is deemed medically beneficial, then the rationing decision is about how to weigh this medical benefit against those of other beneficial treatments competing for the same limited resource. The equal right of all patients with the same condition to receive the same amount of the same treatment is presupposed, whatever that amount may turn out to be in the agreed rationing scheme. Rationing by age, by contrast, would accept that two patients with the same condition might have different priorities for the same treatment because one was young and one was old.

This point may be clearer if we take a specific example, that of the allocation of kidney dialysis. In the first sort of rationing, the question might be what priority should be given to this form of treatment for kidney disease as opposed to treatments for other diseases. The arguments used would concern such things as the amount of human suffering which would be relieved by providing kidney dialysis (in terms both of the numbers of sufferers who would be helped and the intensity of their suffering), in comparison with the competitor treatments and conditions, the comparative costs of achieving the same benefit in the different cases, and so on. In considering age-based rationing, on the other hand, the question would be whether the needs of older people with kidney disease should count as much as, or more than or less than, those of younger people with the same condition. Kidney disease presumably causes the same kind and intensity of suffering and incapacity in a 70-year-old as in a 35-year-old, but the question which is raised is whether there is some reason for thinking that we ought to pay less attention to that suffering and incapacity in the one case than in the other. And similar arguments could in principle apply as much to other treatments for other conditions as to the particular case of kidney dialysis.

All this indicates the kind of argument that would be needed in order to make out a case for age-based rationing. It would have to show that there is something about being old (or being young) which is relevant to the amount, or (perhaps more plausibly) the *kind*, of attention which ought to be paid to the medical conditions of old (young) people. Sexists and racists have, of course, tried unsuccessfully to show that we ought to pay less attention to the suffering of people of one gender, or one skin colour, than to those of another. Their lack of success has been largely due to the sheer implausibility, to any rational person, of the claim that there is anything relevant to this discrimination about being male or female, or black or white. It is not so obviously implausible that there might be something relevant about being old or young. One way to try to make it plausible would be by arguing that the view that there is *nothing* relevant from this point of view about age leads to consequences that any rational person could see to be unacceptable. This is the structure of the argument put forward by Daniel Callahan, which we shall critically examine in the next chapter.

Chapter 7

Callahan and the significance of age

Introduction

There will be an ethical crisis in the NHS if the changing age balance in the population creates insuperable problems of justice or fairness between the younger and the older generation. But if it can be shown that, even in the envisaged demographic situation, a fair system of rationing can be established that takes account of the influence of age – that is, one which respects the genuine *rights* or moral entitlements of both young and old – then the ethical crisis at least is avoidable. What is needed is to show that this is an argument to the effect that the genuine medical *needs* of old people as such are not so great as to impose a morally intolerable burden on younger taxpayers. This in turn requires a consideration of the nature and significance of old age, and, in the light of that, which of the *demands* that older people may currently make on medical services are *needs* which morally require to be satisfied, and which are mere wants, with no special moral claim on resources (cf. the discussion of the difference between demand and medical need in Chapter 2).

One author who has devoted considerable thought to these questions and who has come up with some extremely subtle and provocative answers to them – answers which have generated an extensive literature of both critical and supportive comment – is the distinguished US bioethicist Daniel Callahan. Callahan was one of the founders, and is now a retired director, of the Hastings Center, which is, in most people's opinion, the foremost bioethics centre, not only in the US but in the world. In the last 20 years or so, in a series of books and articles, he has meditated on the problems facing society, particularly in the US, but in the rest of the developed world also, as a result of an ageing population. There is a paucity of works which engage with these problems, at least at a *philosophical* level, and in this literature Callahan's writings tower above the rest in their quality; this is our justification for focusing primarily on his work and the response to it. Callahan sees the ageing of the population as creating problems for our whole understanding of the role of medicine and its relation to society. He writes, naturally, with an eye mainly to *American* society, its values and its system of medical provision, so that one of our tasks will be to see how far, if at all, his arguments and conclusions apply to European systems, and above all to the NHS. But it would be impossible to ignore Callahan's views in any discussion of the alleged 'impending crisis of ageing'. As in earlier chapters, we shall first set out Callahan's arguments as fairly as possible, without criticism, although sometimes we shall point forward to our later critique. Apart from these forward references, however, the views expressed in the following section will be Callahan's, not our own.

Two views of ageing

At the heart of Callahan's position, as was said above, is the view that the increasing proportion of older people in the population calls into question the whole direction which Western medicine and society have taken up to now:

- in respect of the priority given to medical care needs as opposed to other elements of the good society
- in respect of the tendency to see the goal of medicine as being 'to conquer all disease and extend all life'
- in respect of its excessive concern with the individual, rather than the communal, good (Callahan, 1990, Chapter 1).

All of these tendencies are, he accepts, particularly marked in US medicine, but he would contend that they are also to be found, if perhaps less obviously, in Western society generally. The ageing of the population calls them into question, he argues, because the survival of more and more people to an age well beyond the previous average lifespan makes it seem less obvious that medicine ought to be concerned with indefinite extension of the length of life or with the conquest of all medical ills. Another way of expressing this would be to say that it forces us to re-examine our whole way of thinking about the significance of old age and the role played by medicine in dealing with the problems of old age.

Callahan distinguishes two opposing ways of thinking of ageing from a medical perspective. In modern Western society, while we recognise, at least intellectually, that life has certain necessary limits and that, if we survive the contingencies of early life, we must all eventually age and die, we tend not to be:

> prepared to accept those hard truths without a struggle: without first – through the agency of medicine – stretching those limits as if they were not there; and then – through the redefinition of old age as an open frontier and not a closed boundary – all but denying there must be limits (Callahan, 1987, p. 202).

The view of old age which 'all but denies there must be limits' is what Callahan sometimes calls 'the modernisation of ageing' (*see* e.g. Callahan, 1987, p. 26). It is the view that old age is not a special phase of life, the last phase before natural death, and therefore is not essentially different in character and needs from earlier and more physically and mentally vigorous phases. On the 'modernised' view, if older people in fact experience a decline in physical and mental vigour, this is not an *inevitable* consequence of their age (part of the nature of old age as such), but a deficiency to be corrected as far as possible, just as it would be if a younger person became less active as a result of disease. Indeed, this view almost sees ageing itself as a kind of disease (or perhaps it would be better to say a complex of different diseases), and hence as something which in principle could be 'cured' by medicine, and which *ought* to be so cured if it became possible to do so.

The development of this modernised view of ageing has been fostered, according to Callahan, by various causes. One of them is the growth of high-technology medicine itself, which has found ways of extending life (and so postponing death) beyond what was previously considered to be possible, and of removing, or at least bypassing, many of the traditional frailties of old age. This has helped to encourage the conception that the aim of medicine, in respect of old age and death, should be to continue to extend life and to find ways of 'curing' the 'disease' of ageing. It would do so, of course, by small incremental steps, in which the particular afflictions of old age (Callahan mentions such examples as osteoporosis, Alzheimer's disease and arthritis) could be overcome; hence another name which Callahan sometimes uses for this view is 'progressive incrementalism' (Callahan, 1995, p. 22). The ideal end-product of this incremental process might be a condition in which older people suffered no more disadvantages than the young, and so could live a life as nearly as possible indistinguishable from that enjoyed by the younger generation. This ideal might be impossible to reach in practice. But what might be more attainable would be what is sometimes expressed in the phrase 'the compression of morbidity', that is, the postponement of the worst of the traditional effects of ageing until the period immediately before death, which period itself becomes increasingly short in duration. The goal of the modernising approach would then be to reduce ageing to a very short phase at the end of life.

However, it is not only the development of medical technology, in Callahan's opinion, which has promoted the modernised view of ageing. The general value-system of Western, and especially US, society has also been an important factor. At the core of this value-system, he contends, is *individualism*, an overriding concern in each individual for his or her own good, rather than with that of society as a whole. In the particular context of medical care, this individualism expresses itself above all as a sense that the aim of medicine ought to be primarily individual wellbeing, where what counts as 'wellbeing' is determined by the satisfaction of the individual's wants. Thus, since most individuals want to live as long as possible, a principal aim of medicine (on this view) ought to be to enable them to go on living, whatever age they have attained so far: as a principal aim, it ought to be pursued at however great a cost. Again, since most individuals want to continue to enjoy youthful levels of activity, a principal aim of medicine ought to be to enable them to do so (once more, whatever the cost). Medicine should aim to make it possible to be as active at 75 as one was at 35. The converse of this is that medicine has failed, on this view, to the extent that it cannot provide the means for prolonging life and youthful activity as long as possible. Callahan sees a further element of the Western value-system here: the assumption that wellbeing at any age (including old age) crucially depends on 'health', however that term may be defined. It is part of what he means by the modernised view of ageing that medical care is indeed 'healthcare', and that the healthcare system ought to be a principal focus of society's organisation and use of resources. (This assertion about the values of modern medicine will be questioned in our critique.)

It was argued in an earlier chapter that the NHS and similar systems have a 'solidaristic' moral base: that they depend on collective altruism and are in this sense the opposite of individualist. Some might feel, therefore, that Callahan's claims about the individualism of the modern Western value-system do not apply to Britain and other European countries. Callahan himself accepts that there are significant differences between the US on the one hand and Canada and Europe on the other, reflected in the nature of the healthcare systems in each case. But he still maintains that in important respects an individualist value-system affects the approach to medical care in all Western countries. The NHS may not be individualist in one sense, namely that it is not a market system, geared to the satisfaction of individual wants, but is based on the idea of medical care as a human right. Nevertheless, it might be said that in UK culture we interpret the right to medical care in a fundamentally individualist fashion, as the entitlement of each individual to enjoy the best available medical care for his or her individual needs. Furthermore, one could argue that in Britain in general, almost to the same extent as in the US, individualist values prevail, so that the aim of medicine is often proclaimed to be the relief of individual pain and suffering, and the prevention of death for individuals, rather than the common good of society as a whole. Certainly, it seems possible to detect significant elements of what Callahan would call the modernised view of ageing in Britain as well as in the US, and it is as plausible to connect them with these features of the value-system in one country as in the other.

The alternative view of old age and its significance described by Callahan is what he calls 'life-cycle traditionalism' (Callahan, 1995, p. 23). This, as its name implies, is held to be the more ancient view. It sees human life as passing through a series of different stages, each with its own characteristics and significance (cf. Shakespeare's 'Seven Ages of Man'). The essence of each phase is defined both in physiological and social terms. Those who hold this view tend to see the lifecycle as somehow natural and biological, so that the sequence of stages is effectively *necessary* for creatures like ourselves. Callahan himself, who, as we shall see, tends to favour this view, sometimes seems to think of it as reflecting a natural process of growth and decay. We shall argue later that there is no reason to think in this way – that the lifecycle view is as much a social construct as the modernising view – but for the moment we must postpone that and other criticisms and return to the task of outlining Callahan's position without comment.

The following might be a typical account of the human lifecycle given by someone who held this view. First might come a stage of *childhood*, marked by physical vulnerability, but also by growth and development; socially, this stage would be the period of preparation for life, in education and training. A later stage might be *adolescence*, including early adulthood. Biologically, this would be the period in which growth and development reach full maturity, and socially that of greatest energy and activity, in which the education and training received in childhood are first put to use in paid employment and the formation of social relationships, including sexual relationships and the foundation of families. Next might come *middle age*, in which the physical energy and activity would begin to decline, but the social and family relationships would be consolidated, leading amongst other things to the production and rearing of a fresh generation of children. Last of all would come *old age*, marked physiologically by an increasingly rapid decline in powers and energy, and increasing vulnerability to illness and injury, and socially by retirement from paid employment and by the opportunity to use one's acquired life experience ('wisdom') in helping younger people to cope with their problems. (This example of a possible lifecycle view is offered, of course, only for purposes of illustration: there is no suggestion that this is the only account that might be given of the course of a human life. The very fact that various such accounts could be given, however, reinforces the claim that all such accounts are social constructs rather than descriptions of biological facts – but that is a point to be returned to later.)

The relevance of this picture to our present concerns is twofold. First, if we accept it, we are also accepting its implication – that old age with its frailties may not usefully be compared to a 'disease', something to be, as it were, 'cured'; but is rather part of the natural cycle of development of a human life, to be distinguished from other phases in that cycle, and respected for what it essentially is rather than assimilated to something which it is not. Old age, on this view, should in other words be simply accepted, rather than fought against. It should not be a matter for regret, but something to be cherished, that old people are nearing the end of their natural lifespan and cannot be as active in many ways as younger people. Secondly, and consequently, the implication of this view is that the aim of medicine in relation to old age should not be to prolong life still further or to preserve or restore levels of activity and ways of living characteristic of youth or middle age. Those who hold this view would strongly reject any idea of human 'wellbeing', especially for older people, as equivalent to, or even largely dependent on, 'health', in the sense of perfect bodily and mental functioning. Medicine is morally required to make its own contribution to human wellbeing, but that contribution, on this view, is the much more limited, but still important, one of relieving avoidable suffering and treating curable diseases so as to achieve a normal lifespan as far as possible. In the case of old people, who by definition have reached an age which is at, or near, or even beyond the normal lifespan, the contribution that medicine can make to wellbeing is reduced still further, to that of reducing pain and distress. In so doing, it will also, on this view, facilitate the special role which older people alone can play in society – as dispensers of wisdom, carers for their grandchildren or other children, and the like.

The two views of the significance of old age which Callahan offers as alternatives are thus supposed to have a direct bearing on the issue of appropriate medical care for older people, and so on what can be described as their 'medical needs', on which their entitlements in a solidaristic system like the NHS are based. On the 'modernising' view, older people have a right to medical care, not only to relieve pain and distress but also to postpone death as long as possible and to fight against the frailties which would otherwise be part of old age. The latter kinds of care are liable to be more expensive, because they are dependent to a significant extent on high-technology medicine, including the development of new drugs. Thus, at least if we follow Callahan's interpretation, the ageing of the population is indeed likely to result in increasing costs for health services, which will inevitably impose a burden on those whose taxes largely fund these services. On the traditional, 'lifecycle', view, on the other hand, the medical needs of older people are much more restricted than those of younger people; like the young and middle aged, they need relief of pain and distress and treatment of curable diseases, but they do not need the more expensive care required to postpone death and 'cure' the frailties of old age itself. As such, an ageing population would be much less likely to impose a burden on the young. Rationing of medical care on the basis of age could be instituted with perfect moral legitimacy, provided it was confined to restricting the access of older people to high-technology life-prolonging and age-defeating medicine, and did not extend to care designed to make their life less painful or uncomfortable.

Much depends, therefore, on which of these views of old age we take. But how can we choose which view to accept? Is it simply a matter of subjective preference, or are there rational arguments for one view rather than the other? Callahan admits that the idea of 'modernising' old age has a strong appeal to most of us. 'Ageing', he says, 'is nowhere wholly welcomed. Its ultimate effects upon the body and often the mind are destructive, and its outcome is death' (Callahan, 1987, p. 26). Another way of putting this might be to say that in many respects ageing *does* have all the appearance of a disease that we would wish to overcome. Furthermore, to use medical technology to 'abolish ageing' (i.e., to remove the frailties of age and prolong youth, or at least middle age) would enable older people to go on living a 'healthy, self-directing, self-realizing, past-transcending life' (op. cit., p. 27), which many in the modern world see as the ideal for anyone, of any age. If it is such an ideal, some would argue, is it not unfairly discriminatory to deny it to older people, if we have the technological means to enable them too to achieve it?

Nevertheless, Callahan firmly rejects the 'modernising' view, as 'fatally flawed' (op. cit., p. 28). He has many reasons for doing so, although his arguments differ both in their structure and in their strength. These arguments will be subjected to critical analysis at a later stage, but we shall here simply present some of his main contentions without comment. First, he cites 'the vast increase in chronic illness' among the elderly as the average lifespan has increased, and the 'intractable poverty' and isolation endured by a significant proportion of older people in modern society. Thus, he suggests that the triumph of the modernising view has certainly not led to an increase in the real wellbeing of older people, but rather to a decline in their quality of life. The modernisation project, according to Callahan, has also failed to provide any sense of meaning for old age, any purpose to be served by the increased freedom and longer life which old people are supposed to enjoy. To have more years of life, he argues, is not to enjoy greater 'self-realisation' if there is no clear sense of what this self-realisation is supposed to consist of: wellbeing is still further reduced by the disappointment at the failure of the promises of modernisation.

Callahan's objections to modernisation

We shall concentrate, however, on what is undoubtedly Callahan's key objection to the modernisers' position – 'key', both in the sense of being most important to Callahan himself and of being most relevant to our present themes. This is the argument that the modernising view must be rejected because it generates unsustainable costs for the medical care system in particular through inflating everyone's conception of what can or ought to be expected from medicine, and particularly what medicine can or ought to do in relation to old age.

In his 1990 book, Callahan argues that Western medicine has reached the limits of desirable progress, and claims a connection between this assertion and the ageing of the population. The connection seems to be that medical 'progress' has come to be identified, in Western culture, with an increased ability to extend the average length of human life, by using increasingly sophisticated medical technology to 'cure' conditions in earlier life which would previously have been fatal at that stage. 'Cure' is here placed in inverted commas because part of what Callahan seems to be saying is that the relief from the condition is only temporary. Death has not been prevented, only postponed: those who have been 'cured' will be subject at a later stage in their life to all the problems of old age. But because of the prevailing conception of medical progress they will then, in Callahan's view, expect to have their life prolonged still further (or, putting it the other way around, to have death postponed yet again). Thus, he says:

> The larger the number of people saved by acute, high-technology medicine, the larger the number of those who are going to bear some disability and require ongoing acute care and rehabilitation. That process in turn stimulates the need for even more technology, to improve the lives now extended (Callahan, 1990, p. 81).

In this way, he would argue, we have come in the West to believe that we are making medical progress when we find new ways to extend the length of life and to enhance its quality, no matter what the age of the patients in question. If so, then technological progress in medicine has been a major (perhaps *the* major) factor in undermining traditional conceptions of old age as a period of inevitable decline, which we must simply make the best of. Instead, it has created the idea that it is our *right* to have a 'modernised' old age, in which death is postponed as long as possible, and to have all the assistance of medical technology in order to achieve it, at whatever cost.

The result of this conception of medical progress has been, in Callahan's opinion, the creation of three 'insuperable obstacles' to a satisfactory definition of what is to count as adequate medical care. First, he claims, it involves an implicit denial that there are any limits to what is possible, so that standards of adequacy are raised in unreasonable ways. An example, which can be claimed to be in the spirit of what Callahan is saying, though it is not directly derived from him, might be the following case: if there are assumed to be no limits to the possibility of a *desirable* extension of human life, then it becomes merely arbitrary to say, at any particular point, that all the medical effort which is morally required has been made to save a patient's life. In general, on this conception, it is impossible to say that 'adequate' care means all the care that is required to restore normal human functioning if we have no clear idea of what constitutes normal human functioning. For example, if we ought to be continually seeking to enhance the possibilities of life for everyone, irrespective of their age, then there can be no point at which we can say that we have done all that is morally required to improve a person's quality of life, whether that person is young or old.

Secondly, Callahan argues, if there are no fixed limits to what counts as normal human functioning, then the gap between individual needs is widened. Some patients will need much more expensive and sophisticated treatment to reach this constantly receding standard, so that we shall have to accept a widening gap between the treatments given to the former group and those given to the latter.

Thirdly, medical progress understood in this way turns what used to be seen as, at most, *aspirations* into perceived *needs*, thus raising expectations and blurring the gap between what individuals *want* and what they *have a right to*. If we thought of medical care as an ordinary consumer good, of which individuals could have as much as they wanted and could afford, then the moral problem would not arise. But if we think, as is implicit in the very nature of such systems as the NHS, of medical care as a human *right*, something to which human beings are *morally entitled*, then there has to be a clear conception of what constitutes normal functioning for any human being whatsoever, independently of their individual wishes, in order to determine the limits of that entitlement.

Callahan's objection to this idea of medical progress, as a consequence of the modernising view of age, is also his crucial reason for rejecting the modernising view itself. Because it makes it impossible to set limits to the definition of adequate care, he argues, it leads to spiralling and uncontrollable medical care costs, since the removal of any basis for comparing the relative benefits of different sorts of treatment for different sorts of people makes it impossible to apply cost-benefit analysis. This is a *moral* issue, since it concerns justice – a just allocation of medical resources between different individuals and different categories of patients depends essentially on such a comparison of costs and benefits. What particularly concerns us here, of course, is the relative allocation of resources between categories defined by age. Callahan's point in this connection is that, to the extent that medical progress (as seen in Western culture) has removed any concept of possible limits to the prolongation of human life and to overcoming the frailties of old age, it makes it impossible to set limits to the justifiable costs of medical provision for older people. In the long run, he concludes, this would lead to an unsustainable situation (a 'crisis', in our terms), since resources are finite. The fact that it would have this consequence is a prime reason, in his view, for doubting the view of old age which gives rise to it.

If this is Callahan's diagnosis of the nature of the crisis, and his account of its aetiology, what is his proposed treatment? Essentially, since he sees the source of the problem as a misguided conception of the role of medicine, which is in turn part of a misguided value-system in Western culture generally, his suggestion is that the way to avoid crisis is a change in the culture, which would in turn have practical consequences for the system of providing medical care. What are these changes in the culture that he proposes? First, he argues, Western (but especially US) culture has attached too much importance to health and to medical care as conditions for the good life, in comparison with other important human goods. We need, in his view, to think of the good life, especially for older people, as less dependent on the level of one's bodily health. This would in turn mean attaching less importance than we currently do to medical care as a means of achieving a good life. (This goes along, we might add, with the use of the expression 'healthcare', rather than 'medical care': the former expression, as we suggested in the Preface, embodies a view of the role of medicine as not simply the relief of pain and distress but the positive enhancement of human wellbeing.) Secondly, Western culture needs to become less individualist, less concerned with individuals in isolation from other individuals. Such individualism, in his view, is connected with the obsession with health. The good life is seen by each individual as consisting of *their own* wellbeing, of which 'health' in a positive sense is likely to be a major component. If on the other hand we conceive of human beings as above all *social*, not living in isolation but as part of a community, in which they have relationships with other individuals, then, Callahan argues, we are more likely to stress the wellbeing of the community as a whole and to concentrate on collective goods (his examples are such things as schools, roads, houses, parks, police, fire service, etc.). Taking a more communitarian view in this way would thus imply a smaller share of the national income devoted to medical care (or at least no increase in it) and proportionately greater attention to the other sorts of social good just mentioned.

This would have important practical consequences for expenditure on medical care. If we accept Callahan's communitarian view, then, the basis for allocating collective resources ought to be the contribution to general welfare rather than to the wellbeing of individuals as such. In respect of medical care, that would mean that resources were applied so as to maximise the benefit to society as a whole.

Individual wellbeing would feature only in so far as it concerned the ability of individuals to make their own appropriate contributions to the common good. A life in which one made one's own contribution would be, as Callahan expresses it, a 'decent' life, a life of dignity, worthy of respect. The right to medical care would extend to treatment designed to relieve pain and disability which might prevent someone's making their contribution to the common good, but not to that which did no more than enhance the individual's quality of life for its own sake. For older people, this would mean that they would be entitled to such medical care as would enable them to make the special contribution which only they can make, and so achieve the special respect which is owing to them as old people. This would *not*, therefore, be medical care which enabled them to gain more years than their natural span, or which enabled them to live in the ways that are more appropriate to younger people. Callahan therefore envisages a future system of medical provision which would not seek always to overcome all human frailties and decline, but only to help people to cope better with them. His clear assumption is that this would help to bring the costs of medical care under control, so making the system more sustainable and avoiding crisis by, in effect, a system of age-based rationing of medical care.

This is Callahan's solution in broad terms, but what would it amount to in more detail, as far as the care of older members of society is concerned? His proposal is that we should reject the modernising view of old age, which leads to unsustainable and uncontrollable increases in the cost of medical care, and accept instead the more traditional lifecycle view, which enables us to keep medical costs under control. On the lifecycle view, old age has distinct and relevant characteristics of its own. As it is (by definition) the last phase of the lifecycle, it is the period in which bodily functions naturally decline in efficiency, thus increasing vulnerability to disease and injury, but it is also the time in which the accumulated experience of a lifetime can be brought to bear – a time, as it might be expressed, of physical frailty combined with spiritual wisdom. Callahan is perfectly willing to accept that there are individual variations in the rate and extent of decline, but he still wants to insist on increasing frailty as the *essential* feature of old age as such. He is also willing to accept that recent developments in medicine and public health have added some years to the traditional 'threescore years and ten', thus both extending the normal lifespan and postponing the age at which the last phase of life may be thought to begin. This does not, however, in his opinion affect anything crucial in his position. At whatever age in years it may be said to begin – whether 70 or 75 or 80, or even 100 – old age is for him defined as the last phase of life and as the period of decline before death.

As said earlier, Callahan considers that it is one of the undesirable features of modern Western culture that it attaches far too much weight to the achievement of positive health by medical means. But given the alleged special features of old age, he considers that this evaluation of medicine as 'healthcare' is particularly damaging in the culture's view of the lives of old people. If old age is essentially a period of physical decline, then the effort needed to make old people 'healthy' in the positive sense will be all the greater, so that it could be argued that it would be more sensible, and more conducive to the dignity of old age, to keep our medical resources for the more useful purposes of alleviating pain, distress and disability. In this way, medicine will indirectly be having a positive effect:

removing these hindrances to wellbeing will positively enhance old people's lives. His point is rather that there can be no obligation on medicine to contribute in a more obviously 'positive' way, for example by enabling older people to engage in the kind of energetic physical activities which play such an important part in wellbeing for younger people. Good health, for Callahan, is not a necessary condition for happiness at any age, but especially not for old people:

> The goal of the healthcare system should be that of helping us to meet our occupational and social roles and duties while, at the same time, helping us to live effectively within the interpersonal sphere of our lives within communities (Callahan, 1990, p. 115).

In the case of older people, if he is right, this 'social role' is that of helping younger people with the wisdom acquired by longer experience, and of helping parents with the care of children. Old people themselves benefit from this, in Callahan's opinion, because they gain far greater satisfaction, and a far greater sense of self-respect and of usefulness to society, from performing this role than they could ever get from aping the lifestyles of younger people.

Central to Callahan's objection to the modernising view of old age, as we saw, is the claim that it makes it impossible to define any standard of adequacy for medical care of older people. His preferred lifecycle view, by contrast, is held to offer the possibility of such a definition:

> . . . the health of the elderly is adequate when a large majority are able to live out an adequate biographical lifespan (late seventies or early eighties) and are able to carry out interpersonal and community activities of a common type (Callahan, 1990, p. 130).

The acceptability of this definition of adequacy depends in part on whether he has a non-arbitrary basis for his conception of what counts as 'an adequate biographical lifespan'. The basis, as he argues elsewhere, is that a life of this kind of length is sufficient to enable someone to achieve most of their life goals to a reasonable extent and to have had most of the experiences which give value to life. We shall return to the question of whether this basis is indeed non-arbitrary in our own critique, but for the moment let us concentrate on its implications for medical care. One important implication is that there can be no *right* to medical care which would have the primary purpose of extending life *beyond* that adequate limit. The basis for rights to medical care, on Callahan's view, can only be the contribution which such care makes, not to the satisfaction of the preferences of the individual patient, but to the common good of society, and;

> It is not evident . . . that a general increase in life-expectancy (from, say, the present seventy-five years to eighty-five) would make any significant contribution to the overall welfare of society (Callahan, 1990, p. 128).

This would mean, not only that patients had no entitlement to provision of such life-extending care, but that there was no moral obligation to put resources into research on such life-extending treatment.

What about the chronic illnesses which cause so much misery to those who suffer from them, and which in many cases are so particularly associated with old age? Callahan gives as examples Alzheimer's disease, cancer, stroke, heart disease and multi-organ failure (he also mentions schizophrenia, but only as an instance of a chronic disorder, without suggesting that it is typically a disease of old age). His first point about such conditions is that they are not, for the most part, threats to the population as a whole, but tend to be affected by such individual features as genetic inheritance. Secondly, he argues that, because of the correlation with ageing, the only consequence of any attempt to reduce or eradicate such conditions by medical means will be that new conditions of the same sort will emerge to replace them. This means that research on treatments for them will be both costly and likely to be futile. The conclusion drawn is that it is 'morally optional' for society whether it tries to eliminate such conditions, i.e. to develop cures for them. To attempt to do so would result in even higher costs, which would be morally questionable in relation to the expected benefits:

> A society cannot be said to owe its citizens the pursuit of every medical possibility to meet every curative need, much less when the possibilities of doing so are endless (Callahan, 1990, p. 138).

What is not 'morally optional', however, is that society must provide *care* for individuals afflicted with such conditions, that is, must alleviate the associated pain and distress and help them to cope as well as possible with the consequences of the condition, including death.

This brings us to one of Callahan's central moral distinctions, between 'caring' and 'curing'. A system of medical provision which is to ensure the decent functioning of society, he says, must be one based on 'our mutual and shared response to the suffering of others' (Callahan, 1990, p. 141). What disturbs us most as decent human beings, he argues, is the suffering of our fellow human beings. We can empathise with it, because all human beings necessarily see suffering as an evil, something to be avoided. Deprivation of other goods, which affects different people differently, is for that very reason harder to empathise with. By 'suffering' in this context, Callahan means 'a sense of anguish, vulnerability, loss of control, and threat to the integrity of the self'. 'Caring' can then be defined as:

> a positive emotional and supportive response to the condition and situation of another person, a response whose purpose is to affirm our commitment to their well-being, our willingness to identify with them in their pain and suffering, and our desire to do what we can to relieve their situation (Callahan, 1990, p. 144).

'Caring' is thus the simple relief of suffering, as opposed to 'curing', by which he seems to mean the attempt to restore someone to positive health. The priority of caring over curing, for him, results both from its centrality to what we mean by human decency and from the fact that caring, unlike curing, is something which individuals, and the medical system as a whole, can almost always offer to everyone. Because it depends to a large extent, not on expensive technology, but on simple human attributes of sympathy and concern, caring makes it possible to contain costs while yet meeting a clear moral demand in our dealings with each other. In practice, making caring central to our provision for older people means providing such structures as hospices for the dying, home care programmes (where feasible) or otherwise institutional care, legal and social work assistance, community services, etc.

The priority of care over cure does not, however, in Callahan's view, mean that there should be no place at all for curative medicine, only that limits to it need to be accepted. These limits should be based, first, on recognition of the finitude of the human body, that is, the inevitability of death, ageing and illness (cf. Callahan, 1990, p. 151). Thus, we can allow the use of medical and surgical treatment to prolong life to a 'reasonable' extent, by which Callahan means, up to his 'adequate' lifespan (up to the early 80s). Other acceptable goals for curative medicine in old age would, in his view, include the creation of a psychologically stable mental and emotional state and of a state of adequate functional capacity for a person of the relevant age. But these other goals, he contends, are to be regarded only as 'aspirations', not targets to be met in each individual case. Curative technologies should be prioritised, not according to some mechanical formula, but on the basis of general principles of judgement, guided by the need to limit costs rather than by 'bright visions of progress'. We should balance the extension of the quantity of life against the improvement of its quality (the 'principle of symmetry'). For instance, we should use technology primarily to relieve the suffering of those who have already survived, rather than devising new technologies to make survival possible in new kinds of cases. And we should judge medical technologies by two criteria:

* Do they achieve well their stated medical purpose?
* Would their widespread use tend to produce distortions in the system, 'especially that of threatening societally necessary limits on the frontiers of ageing and individual need' (Callahan, 1990, p. 167). (This he calls 'the principle of technology assessment'.)

On this basis, Callahan argues for the necessity of change at three levels if we are to avoid a crisis.

* At the *cultural* level (the values of our way of life), we need to change our view that positive health is a major component of human wellbeing. We should see it, rather, simply as a means to an end, to be valued only to the extent that it contributes to individual flourishing and social welfare. That means, among other things, an acceptance of ageing, sickness, decline and death as a necessary part of the human condition, and the primary role of medicine as being simply that of alleviating them.
* At the level of *entitlement* (our views about rights to healthcare), we need to see justice in the medical context as consisting of a system which provides everyone, from collective resources, with a guaranteed minimum level of medical care (with the emphasis on 'caring' rather than 'curing'). Individuals and employers would then be free to agree benefit packages above the minimum for those willing to pay for them from their own resources. (In the British situation, that would mean that the NHS provided the guaranteed minimum for everyone, while medical care above that minimum would be provided by private insurance for those who could afford it.)

- At the *institutional* level (the institutions by which medical care is provided), the change would be a restriction on individual freedom of choice, on the grounds of justice. This would in turn require a great degree of central planning and organisation.

This third change would be most marked in the US system, since it is already an integral part of the NHS that allocation decisions are made centrally, on the grounds of justice and cost-containment rather than of meeting consumer preferences. However, the kind of two-tier system envisaged by Callahan might well require an even greater degree of central planning than presently exists in the NHS.

Before proceeding in the next chapter to critical analysis, we can usefully conclude the present chapter with a brief summary of the main features of Callahan's position. He sees Western medicine as descending further and further into crisis because it is an essential part of Western culture, with its high valuation of the importance of individual physical wellbeing, and its conception of medical progress as consisting of the development of new forms of technology to promote such wellbeing. This leads, in his opinion, to unlimited demands to enjoy the fruits of medical progress in this sense, and so to uncontrollable medical costs which are both unsustainable in themselves and which also compete with expenditure on other kinds of social goods, such as education, roads, and other kinds of public services. This general crisis of Western culture and of Western medicine can be seen as a crisis of ageing in particular for three main reasons.

- The costs of achieving positive health are necessarily greater in the case of older people, because the obstacles to health to be overcome are greater in their case.
- Partly as a result of medical progress, the numbers of older people in the population are increasing.
- There are problems of intergenerational justice involved, since many of the other social goods with which increased medical expenditure competes particularly benefit younger people (e.g. education, unemployment benefit, etc.).

Callahan sees this crisis of ageing as avoidable, if we limit our expectations of what medicine can contribute to our wellbeing, especially in our later years. In effect, he wants to change the perceptions of what we *need* medically, and so of what our *rights* or entitlements are in this respect. This would make it possible both to contain overall medical costs (for everyone) to a much more sustainable level and in particular to introduce age-based rationing, at least of curative medicine, without infringing on justice and human rights. In the next chapter, we shall examine these contentions in a more critical spirit.

Chapter 8

A critique of Callahan

Introduction

Callahan's dissection of the problems created by 'a world growing old' is subtle, original and thought provoking; we cannot fail to learn from it, even from those respects in which we may disagree with Callahan. His analysis embodies feelings about the current situation which have been expressed, although perhaps less clearly and systematically, by others, and which have contributed to the perception of crisis. In the early part of Chapter 1 we looked at some expressions of this from as far back as the 1930s. By a critical analysis of his views, drawing partly on this literature and partly on our own discussions, we believe we can make some progress in our own understanding of the 'perceived crisis of ageing' and its implications for ethics and policy. This is what we shall attempt to do in this chapter. Our critical examination will need to focus both on Callahan's diagnosis of the causes of possible crisis and on his proposed solution, though these aspects of his analysis cannot ultimately be considered separately.

Does Callahan ask the right questions?

Callahan sees the crisis as fundamentally one facing modern Western culture as a whole, though the most relevant aspect of that culture from this point of view is its attitude towards medicine and its role in contributing to human welfare. In modern Western societies, his claim is that welfare has been interpreted primarily in terms of *individual* wellbeing, in the sense of an increased enjoyment of life free from pain, vulnerability, fear or discomfort. In this value-system, people are better off when they are able to live longer and to enjoy more pleasurable experiences. Scientific knowledge has provided the basis of technologies, including medical technologies, aimed at making people better off in this sense. Hence, as we saw in the previous chapter, *progress* in medicine has come to be conceived, in Callahan's opinion, as technological advance of this sort. It would indeed be hard to disagree with the contention that the history of modern medicine has been marked by remarkable technological advances, which have contributed to the rise in average lifespan by such things as transplant and bypass surgery, the development of cures for infectious diseases, and so on. By changing people's expectations of what can be done by medicine, these developments have in turn increased the demand for more and more of the same.

As with all technology, these medical advances have in effect liberated human beings from the limitations imposed by nature. In the natural order of things, for example, if an animal is infected by a disease it will probably die, unless it is extremely lucky. By curing such infections, medicine frees the human animal from the natural order. The particular manifestation of this on which Callahan concentrates, because he seems to see it as the heart of the crisis in medicine, is human liberation from the process of ageing and death (or, rather, in his view, the *idea* that such a liberation might become possible through further medical advance, and the attempt to move progressively towards it). This is what he calls, as we saw in the last chapter, the 'modernisation' of ageing. This is the view that increasing frailty in old age is no more inevitable than undergoing all the miseries of an infectious disease. Few, if any, would go so far as to deny the inevitability of death, but many aspire to *postponing* death for as long as possible, so that liberation in this case would be extension of the lifespan.

Medical technology tends to be expensive, so that an increasingly technological medicine is likely to be (and indeed is) more costly. As we have argued already, this would not in itself create a crisis if medical provision were organised on a purely market basis. The normal price mechanisms would control costs, since any medical treatment which was seen as too expensive would price itself out of the market, however much people might wish to have it. The problem arises, in Callahan's view (if we are right in interpreting him this way), in societies in which people believe they have a *right* to medical care, because such care is not a commodity, to be bought and sold according to customers' ability to pay, but a human need of the kind that they are morally entitled to have satisfied. Once this is accepted, and given this view of the purpose of medicine, then costs, in Callahan's view, become effectively uncontrollable. If it is a universal right to have medical care, then it must be supplied to everyone who requires it, whatever the cost. There is a potential crisis of ageing, according to Callahan, not only because of the increasing numbers of older people, living to greater and greater ages, but also because those old people consider they have a human right to be freed from the frailties of age and to have even longer lives. As we have seen, Callahan's proposed solution to the crisis, or perhaps better his way of avoiding a crisis, is to lower general expectations of the benefits to be achieved by medicine, and above all to restore a more traditional perception of old age and its needs so as to reduce expenditure on medical care both for prolonging and for improving the quality of the lives of older people.

If expensive technological treatment is not a genuine *need* in old age, then no human rights will be infringed in denying it to older people, and so no problems of justice will arise. What is important in the context of this book is that, strictly speaking, what he is proposing is not so much an imposed system of rationing based on age, but a change in the climate of opinion such that people would ration *themselves* on the basis of age, or would at least willingly accept age-based rationing of medical care.

The first critical question about Callahan's argument is whether his attribution of the alleged crisis as caused by a crisis of *ageing* is correct. This is not really a single question, but a complex of different questions which must as far as possible be disentangled. Callahan conflates a number of issues that are arguably distinct from each other and ought to be treated separately. There is, for instance, the issue of the nature of modern medicine and the value-system that underpins it. There is also the claim that attitudes to ageing have changed, and the associated claim that modern conceptions of old age are in some way 'worse' than the more traditional view. There is the question of whether the demand for medical care allegedly generated by the modernised conception of old age is the major contributor to a crisis of uncontrollable costs facing modern medicine. And there is the question of whether, if what is said in the previous sentence is correct, this constitutes a *moral* argument against the modernised conception of old age and in favour of the introduction of age-based rationing of medical services. There may well be other questions raised by Callahan's analysis, but these seem to be the major ones that we must distinguish if we are to see how far, if at all, we can agree with his conclusions.

It is self-evident that modern medicine is increasingly technological. It is also an empirical fact that much 'high-technology' medicine is expensive, at least in its initial stages of development and use, although it should also be said that in some cases medical advance leads to a *reduction* of overall costs, for instance, by cutting down the time which patients need to spend in hospital, by restoring them to normal levels of functioning more quickly, and so on. Many would agree that the rises in the costs of medicine which have led to attempts at cost-containment in many countries are at least to some extent due to the increasing use of expensive methods of treatment and diagnosis which are 'technological' in a broad sense, but include the development of new drugs and the introduction of new types of surgery as well as the use of shiny machinery. The increasingly technological character of medicine, it can also be agreed, is a response to demands inspired by the value-system which currently prevails in post-Enlightenment Western societies. People expect technology, including medical technology, to free them from the limitations imposed by nature so that they can lead increasingly autonomous lives devoted to the pursuit of their own aims. If a vaccine, for instance, can prevent someone catching a disease which they would otherwise have been very likely to catch, and which would have killed them or seriously disabled them, then they can be freed from that fear and liberated to that extent to pursue the pattern of life which they choose for themselves.

One of the limitations which nature imposes on all human beings is that they will eventually die and, in earlier times, the average age of death was much lower than in the modern Western world. For those lucky enough to survive beyond, traditionally, about 60 years of age, nature has imposed a further limitation – that in most cases they will become increasingly frail and vulnerable and will experience a slow (or not so slow) decline in their physical and mental powers until death. In our discussion in Chapter 2 we agreed with Callahan that these limitations too have to some extent been overcome in modern Western society, and in part through advances in medical technology. The average life expectancy is greater now than in the past, and since the 1980s some of the increase has been in people aged 65 or more. The latter has been due to a combination of medical advances and greater fitness of those who reach that age. In general, however, that greater fitness and the overall improvement in length of life is as much a result of reductions in infant mortality and of improvements in social conditions and in nutrition as of the kind of technological interventions in curing disease which Callahan emphasises. It is noteworthy that there is still a wide variation in lifespan between people from more privileged social classes, who have enjoyed more of the benefits of good nutrition and healthy living conditions, and those from a more deprived background. Nevertheless, it can be accepted that medical advances in treating otherwise life-threatening diseases in earlier life clearly mean that more people survive to old age than was previously the case. Equally, as was also said in Chapter 2, retired people now very often enjoy higher levels of activity and a generally much better quality of life than they did even a generation or two ago. Old age is not necessarily as much of an affliction in itself as in the past. Here again, this is partly due to improved social conditions and nutrition throughout life, as indicated by the fact that the more affluent still tend to enjoy more active lives in old age than those with smaller incomes. Some improvements are, however, due to medical advance. We may think, for instance, of the increased mobility for arthritis sufferers (typically older people) resulting from hip and knee replacements. And people of any age, including older people, may wish to enjoy the benefits of the kinds of curative treatment for disease made possible by modern technology.

All this can be accepted, but the conclusions that Callahan draws will follow only if he can give appropriate answers to certain pertinent questions. First, is it in fact the case that the demand for such expensive high-technology treatments to overcome the allegedly natural limitations *specifically of old age* has made a disproportionate contribution to the spiralling in the costs of medical care, and will, unless regulated, make those costs uncontrollable? This is an empirical, factual, question, and the evidence cited in Chapter 2 suggests that it is at least doubtful whether the ageing of the population and the demand for high-technology medicine for older people has made any significant extra contribution to overall costs; and it is more than doubtful therefore that it will lead to *uncontrollable* costs in the future. But Callahan associates this empirical question with another question which is essentially ethical. If the application of high-technology medicine, in extending the length as well as improving the quality of life for *older* people, makes any significant contribution to an increase in costs for the medical care system, ought we to restrict that application in the interests of justice? After all, if there is nothing special about older people in this respect, then the way to control increased costs resulting from the use of high-technology medicine ought surely to be to restrict that use *for everyone*. The just answer to the spiralling costs of high-technology medicine is to ration it according to need, and it is only if it can be shown that the needs of older people are less worthy of attention (and less worthy just because they are old) that age ought to function as a rationing criterion.

How good are Callahan's answers?

So what kinds of answer to this second, moral, question can be found in Callahan's writings? Sometimes, he appears to be saying simply that the traditional lifecycle account, in which the demands made on medicine by older people are restricted, is superior to the modernisation of ageing because it is 'natural'. But there are various objections to this argument, if it can be dignified with that term. First, it is a commonplace of modern moral philosophy that to say something is more 'natural', in the sense of not resulting from conscious human intervention, is never a reason for saying it is morally superior. It is more 'natural' in that sense not to wear clothes, or to live in houses, or to cook food, but no one would say it follows from that fact that nudity or living in the open air or eating raw food are morally superior. More pertinently, medical care, as said earlier, has long been devoted to defying nature. To cure a disease is necessarily to interfere with 'nature' in this sense, and so far from thinking this makes it morally unacceptable, we give moral approval to someone who saves a life in this way.

The use of medicine to defy nature, and the idea that it is a good thing to do, is certainly not a product of the recent development of high-technology medicine. Modern medicine differs only in that it now has the means to be more successful in fulfilling that aim. What Callahan needs to show is why saving (extending) a life is morally approvable in other cases but not in that of someone over 80.

Secondly, as we suggested in the last chapter, it is questionable whether the lifespan account which Callahan offers is in accord with nature, in the sense of reflecting the unalterable biological course of a human life. The very fact, as was said then, of the variations in accounts of the lifecycle between individuals and cultures indicates that the lifecycle account is a social construction rather than the reflection of an inescapable natural sequence. It may, in its broad outlines, be 'traditional' in our culture (and perhaps in most others) and every bit as valid as a biological definition, but that in itself gives us no more reason for accepting it than we have for accepting any other traditional view, such as the tradition of regarding women as naturally inferior to men. Furthermore, many recent biologists have questioned the biological inevitability of ageing. For instance, the leading gerontologist Tom Kirkwood, in his 2001 Reith Lectures, says categorically, 'Science has new things to tell us about the process of ageing. Now we know that ageing is no longer inevitable or necessary' (Kirkwood, 2001, p. 3). Kirkwood rejects the theory that we are genetically pre-programmed to age and die. Among other arguments, he points to other species 'that manage the amazing feat of living indefinitely without intrinsic deterioration' (Kirkwood, 2001, p. 10). Other scientists, like William R Clark, Professor Emeritus of Immunology at UCLA, dispute this kind of argument, and consider that 'There is every reason to believe that ageing – senescence – is under genetic control' (Clark, 1999, p. 190). But this does not lead him, any more than Kirkwood, to believe that there is nothing that can be done technologically to alleviate the traditionally expected effects of ageing and to extend the lifespan beyond what it is at present. Callahan himself, as we have seen, is prepared to adjust the traditional picture at least to the extent of accepting the increases in average lifespan already achieved, which in itself implies that the length of life someone can expect is to some extent manipulable by human action. If so, then it is hard to see why we should accept, at any rate without further argument, a traditional view of the lifecycle as defining what is morally permissible. (In addition, Callahan is open to criticism for his apparent equation of the *lifecycle* view with a particular conception of a desirable human *lifespan*: one could perfectly logically accept the lifecycle approach while allowing for the continuing indirectly achieved increase in life expectancy after 65.)

At the end of the day, Callahan's defence of the traditional lifecycle view depends solely on the *costs* allegedly created by modernised expectations about ageing. This is where he finds the further argument required – the use of resources to overcome ageing and to extend life further than it has already been done, even if it became technically possible, would be morally objectionable because it would be unfair to younger people. Why would that be so? One argument is that younger people should take priority in the case of life-extending medical technology on the grounds that they would benefit more from it in both quantity and quality of life-years gained. (This kind of argument is supported by Alan Williams (Williams, 1997)). For instance, it might be said that young people cured of life-threatening diseases by expensive technology would live longer afterwards and each of these extra years of life would have greater quality. The familiar concept of the quality-adjusted life year (QALY) might be thought to favour this line of thinking, since the cost per QALY would clearly be reduced, even for expensive treatments, if the numbers of QALYs gained were increased. (Interestingly, some have criticised the QALY concept for this reason as 'ageist': for example, Harris, 1988). One strength of this argument is that it does not depend on any mere speculation about possible 'natural limits' to human life, but only on the undeniable fact that we must all die sometime, and the logical consequence that those who have already lived longer are likely to have fewer years left than those who are younger.

It has, however, been suggested that there is also a weakness in this argument, in that it is not necessarily the case that a person of, say, 75 will live fewer years after a successful life-prolonging treatment than someone of, say, 45. For example, one of Callahan's US critics, Christine Cassel, says:

> [Callahan's] first mistake is to assume that at age eighty or eighty-five so little potential benefit can be gained from medical care that few months or years of remaining life would be lost by an arbitrary cut-off of life-sustaining or life-extending medical treatment at that point (Cassel, 1999, p. 659).

She refers to current demographic studies which suggest that lifespan itself may be increasing, and concludes that 'Treatment of a life-threatening illness in an 85-year-old could save 10 or 15 years of life', which could, she argues, be life of high quality even in an 'objective' sense, and enable the person to make a useful contribution to society. Callahan himself allows that older people can make a useful contribution to society, even if not primarily in the sense of being economically productive, but in that of communicating their experience and wisdom, helping with child-rearing, and so on. Cassel, however, seems to be factually mistaken herself about the effectiveness of therapies in older people and it is misguided to base moral arguments on dubious factual claims.

Callahan and the value of human life

But there is a much deeper issue raised by Callahan's argument, and it may be that this is what Cassel is really trying to express in this misleading form. In a joint article which Cassel wrote with Bernice Neugarten, this deeper issue is expressed in these words:

> Such statements [as Callahan's] raise fundamental moral questions about the value of human life (Cassel and Neugarten, 1994, p. 96).

The way in which these fundamental moral questions are raised is made clear by Cassel (Cassel, 1999), where Cassel argues that Callahan's view rests on the assumption that it would be fairer (to the younger generation) to have an arbitrary cut-off point at a certain age, at which all medical care was withdrawn from patients, rather than to continue as at present (by which she presumably means trying to balance medical expenditure between older and younger people). This would, she claims, have 'draconian' consequences, resulting 'precipitously in five million deaths' (Cassel, 1999, p. 659) (the figure of five million refers to the number of people currently over 80 years of age, presumably, although Cassel does not make this clear, in the US). If this were a consequence of Callahan's position, then adopting his proposals would indeed, as she says, drastically undermine society's respect for older people, and ultimately for human life generally. For it would mean, not only that younger people have a right to a life equal to that of older people, but also that older people, simply as such, have no right to continued life in their last years. That in turn would imply that different human beings can have different worth, simply on the basis of the number of years they have been alive: so that it is not human life itself which is valued, but the life of vigour and activity which is characteristic of younger people.

Callahan's *explicit* position does not seem open to this objection. He says, as we have seen, that there is a moral duty to continue to provide medical *care* for those over 80 (or whatever other age is chosen), and so to keep them alive as long as nature will allow. His objection, he says, is only to the continuation of *curative* medicine, the attempt to use medicine to keep people alive by extraordinary means when their life is threatened by disease; many philosophers would argue that failing to keep someone alive, at least in such circumstances, is morally distinct from actively killing the person. If so, then Callahan's position does not imply that the life of an older person is less worthwhile than that of someone younger, still less that we should actively kill off everyone over 80. It does not even imply that we should allow all over-80s to die immediately. Withdrawal of all access to life-prolonging medicine would not mean immediate death for anyone who was not already near death, and for the latter death would be caused, not by the withdrawal of treatment, but by the disease or injury from which they were already suffering.

Although Callahan himself may be able to find a way round such objections, however, there are other recent writers who have been prepared to be more radical and outspoken in proposing solutions to the crisis of ageing which have at least something in common with Callahan's. For instance, Margaret Pabst Battin (Battin, 1994) argues that in an ageing population age-based rationing of medical care might be required on grounds of fairness to the younger generation. Her argument for this is based on the kinds of considerations advanced by Norman Daniels and already examined in an earlier chapter of the present work. Thus, she says that those under 'an appropriately thin veil of ignorance', and making rational choices about medical provision for someone's life as a whole, 'will know that a given measure of health care is not equally effective at all age ranges; it will be much more effective in younger years, much less effective in old age' (Battin, 1994, p. 63). As she goes on to elaborate, 'by and large, a unit of medical care consumed late in life will have much less effect in preserving life and maintaining normal species-typical function than a unit of medical care consumed at a younger age' (id., ibid.). It will thus be prudent for them, as Daniels argues, to prioritise care for younger people, which will use resources more effectively. The costs of achieving a normal lifespan for a younger person will be less than those involved in achieving a much shorter extension of the length of life beyond the normal limits for someone older. And that use of expenditure will result in a better life overall for everyone, and thus be in accord with justice.

We have already expressed criticisms of Daniels's argument, but for the present let us set them aside in order to consider Battin's position, which draws conclusions from Daniels's argument which go far beyond those reached by Daniels himself. Where Battin goes beyond both Daniels and Callahan is in wishing, on grounds of fairness to younger people in the demographic circumstances envisaged, to deny older people not only elaborate and expensive treatment but, at any rate in certain circumstances, 'a very large proportion of all health-care expenses'. In order to understand the full force of Battin's contentions it is necessary to quote the relevant passage at some length:

> Although allocations to the elderly would, of course, be a fluctuating function of scarcity in health-care resources as a whole, it is probably fair to estimate that were the degree of scarcity approximately equivalent to what it is now, a just distribution of health care would demand that a very large proportion of all health-care expenses now devoted to the elderly be reassigned to younger age groups. Were these resources reassigned to the younger and middle-aged groups, the probability would be dramatically increased that all or virtually all these persons . . . would not only reach a normal lifespan, but reach it in reasonably good health (Battin, 1994, p. 64).

Battin makes it clear in what follows just what kind of reallocation of resources would be required, if a substantial difference is to be made to the prospects of younger people:

> At most, perhaps, minimal home hospice care and inexpensive pain relief could be routinely granted, together with some superficial care in transient acute illness not related to chronic conditions or interdependent diseases. But treatment for the elderly could not be escalated very much beyond this point if, within a fixed degree of scarcity, a just distribution of resources were still to be achieved; . . . (Battin, 1994, p. 65).

She accepts that withdrawal of anything over and above minimal care would result in many earlier deaths, and that it would involve withdrawal of extended medical and nursing care for such conditions as Alzheimer's disease, certain types of arthritis and cancer, osteoporosis or stroke.

This programme would, therefore, be truly 'draconian', to use Cassel's term. Battin accepts that 'the rational self-interest maximiser, behind the veil of ignorance' would be concerned to avoid this consequence of their agreement to a policy of age-based rationing. But the way to avoid it which she proposes is the most controversial aspect of her highly controversial paper. She in effect argues that, given agreement to this kind of reallocation of resources from the old to the young, it would be more humane to accept that those who reach the relevant age should be actively killed *before* their quality of life deteriorates to the point at which they would require the expensive treatment which is to be denied them. To accept a policy which continued one's life while denying any relief of the suffering that would accompany these extra years would not be a choice that a 'rational self-interest maximiser' would make. It would be more rational, Battin argues, to agree that one should undergo euthanasia at the relevant point, especially since this would be a condition for the kind of allocation of medical resources which had enabled one to live to the relevant age. Because of this, there would be a moral pressure on elderly people to end their lives.

Many would see this as a moral *reductio ad absurdum* of the position from which Battin starts, and we shall shortly consider arguments in support of that view. But before discussing that, it is worth noting that Battin could be seen as simply carrying Callahan's views to a logical conclusion, which Callahan himself fails to recognise. Callahan too wants to avoid uncontrollable medical costs arising from the increasing numbers of old people and the culturally-shaped demands made by them by in effect reallocating resources away from the old; but he differs from Battin in that he wants to continue with 'care'. Like Battin, he accepts that we have a moral duty, if we keep people alive, to provide them with care. But unlike Callahan, Battin recognises that this is illogical. What Callahan calls 'care' is itself expensive, so that any cost-savings from the removal of curative treatment would be offset by the costs of medical and nursing care, especially over the long-term. If the only moral imperative is to transfer resources from old to young, then the costs of care should no more be excluded from the reallocation than those of curative treatment.

Thus, Callahan sees the crisis of ageing in essentially the same way as Battin, but refuses to draw her conclusion that the solution to the crisis must involve controlling the costs of 'care' as well as 'cure' for older people. And that would indeed mean, on Callahan's own assumptions, not only that old people were allowed to die earlier for want of a cure, but that their last years should be devoid of all but the most minimal care also, which is contrary to the moral principle which Callahan accepts. There seems only one logical conclusion, and it is the one which Battin draws, namely, that old people should be encouraged to die before they need expensive care to make their lives tolerable. Perhaps, then, Cassel's condemnation of Callahan's proposals as 'draconian', while it may not apply to the proposals as explicitly stated by Callahan, does apply to their logical consequences, to which Callahan seems to have turned a blind eye. If so, then the criticisms that can be made of Battin would apply equally to Callahan.

A forceful critique of what we may call the 'Battin/Callahan' position is provided by the Canadian feminist philosopher Christine Overall (Overall, 2003). Overall first points out that the assumption made by both Callahan and Battin that there is, in Western nations, a situation of scarcity in medical resources is open to question. There is no clear evidence, she says, that Western societies have yet succeeded in achieving a fair distribution and use even of existing resources, and 'Until existing health-care assets are fairly distributed, it is at least premature to make absolute claims about a scarcity of resources' (Overall, 2003, p. 89). But even if there is a scarcity, she argues, it is far from clear that rationing based on age is the only, or the best, way to solve it, particularly if the implication of that rationing policy is that the old should be under severe social pressure to end their lives. 'Any moral and political principles', Overall says:

> that treat elderly or disabled people as if they are social liabilities who must give up the entitlement to go on living and to enjoy life's possibilities are unjust and prejudicial in ways we would never countenance, at the policy level, with respect to other groups (Overall, 2003, pp. 93–4).

The principles in question here are those on which Battin's proposals are based, namely, that policies for resource allocation are those which would be adopted by 'rational self-interest maximisers', operating behind a veil of ignorance, i.e.

making choices independently of any knowledge of how the policies adopted would affect them. Like Daniels, as we have seen, Battin considers that such individuals would choose a distribution over someone's lifetime which ensured that each life, taken as a whole, would maximise that person's self-interest. Again like Daniels, she assumes that that would mean choosing to give preference to a use of resources which would best ensure that one had a chance of living to the normal lifespan, even if that implied withholding resources required for treatment of those ills which afflict people who have lived beyond the normal lifespan.

As we saw when discussing Daniels, however, even if this were the policy which a prudent individual might choose for themselves, it does not follow that it is a *just* policy for the allocation of collective resources, in a system such as the NHS, based on the moral principle of solidarity. The principle of solidarity is not concerned with the maximisation of each person's self-interest over their lifetime as a whole, but with provision to those in most need funded by those best able to pay. It is of course a matter of justice that each person should have an equally good chance of living a life which is satisfactory as a whole; but it does not follow that it is a matter of justice to ensure that the young (at any given time) as a group have a better chance of living to 70 or 80, rather than that those over that age (at the same time) should continue to be cared for and enabled to go on living as long as nature or chance will allow. In a solidaristic system, what should determine the allocation of medical resources is need. The very facts cited by writers like Battin as making old people a 'burden' – their vulnerability and frailty – are evidence that their needs for care are greater, and therefore that their rights to such care ought to be defended, not taken away from them.

The value of older people's lives

This brings us back to the point made by Cassel and Neugarten, that proposals like those of Callahan and Battin raise fundamental moral questions about the value of human life. To say, as Battin does, that the costs of caring for older people and keeping them alive are such a burden on younger people that the older people ought not to be kept alive at all, or, if they go on living, ought not to receive more than the barest minimum of medical care, is to say that an old life is less worth caring for than a young one. Callahan does not appear, on the surface at least, to go that far. He wants old people to continue to receive care, but not curative therapy. But his reason for denying curative therapy to old people is that to provide it will allegedly increase medical costs to an uncontrollable level and will thus create an intolerable burden on the resources of the community as a whole, and above all on the younger members of the community. The implication is that medical expenditure directed towards the treatment of older people, at least when its aim is to prolong their lives, is less morally justifiable than that directed towards those who are younger. In turn, that implies that an old life is less valuable than a young one.

But on what does this alleged difference in value rest? In traditional Western values, a human life is a human life, worthy of equal respect no matter how old the person whose life it is may be. Why should the life of an old person be less worth prolonging than that of a young one? We have already rejected the view that it is because the older person can in the nature of things expect fewer more years of life than the younger. Is it perhaps that the older person has already had a 'good run for their money', whereas the younger person has not? (*See also* Williams, 1997). This seems to be implied by some of Callahan's and Battin's remarks. But although an older person by definition has had more years of life already than the younger person, it by no means follows that every older person has had a better chance to enjoy life or to derive satisfaction from it. In other words, a longer innings is not necessarily a better one (however 'better' is defined) *from the point of view of the 'batsman'*. The chances of a good life (again, however defined) depend much more on social and economic advantage, on natural gifts and the blessing of a good constitution, and on pure good fortune, than on the number of years one has lived. As Christine Overall points out, if the question is posed as one about the justice of using *public* resources on prolonging the lives of those who have already 'had a good innings' rather than on those who have still to play, then that does not address the issue of older people who can use their own *private* resources to keep themselves alive in old age:

> So [she goes on] wealthy persons, who may already have had a full and rewarding life, will be enabled to prolong their lives still further, while poor people, who may have been deprived of many of life's rewards, will be unable to stave off death despite their lack of access to material and social opportunities (Overall, 2003, p. 83).

This hardly sounds to most of us like justice, and that is an indication of the reasons for saying that Battin's conclusion (and implicitly Callahan's) represents a moral *reductio ad absurdum* of the principles from which she starts. There must be something wrong with these principles if they lead to such absurd (in this case, morally unacceptable) conclusions.

The root of what is wrong seems to us to be the same as what was argued in an earlier chapter to be wrong with Daniels's 'Prudential Lifespan Account'. Daniels there, we claimed, confused considerations of *prudence* with those of *justice*. We can now elaborate on this with an eye to what Battin (and implicitly Callahan) are suggesting. Prudence is a matter of sensibly ordering one's dealings (in this case, one's use of medical resources) with a view to maximising one's own long-term self-interest. Thus, an individual choosing a package of medical insurance for herself would prudently choose the one which would produce the best overall pattern of benefits for herself over her lifetime. This might well involve choosing to spend more in her younger years, in order as far as possible to ensure she lived a reasonable number of years, rather than in later years to extend her life beyond that reasonable span. A collectivity, such as a state, in allocating its resources, would behave prudently if it directed them in such a way as to maximise the collective interest. Again, that might well mean giving priority to medical care for younger people, who are still economically productive, rather than on retired people, who have by definition ended their period of economic productivity. In neither case, however, would this *prudent* allocation have anything to do with *justice*. In the individual case, the prudent choice would be directed to producing the best chances of a good life as a whole for the person making the choice. In the collective case, it would be the one which best served the interests of the whole community. In either case, the prudent decision is the one which uses resources in the most cost-effective way.

Justice, however, is not concerned with maximising self-interest, either of the individual or of the whole society, but with getting a certain kind of balance between the *rights* or entitlements of different individuals, so as to create a society which, whether efficient or productive or not, is a good society in *moral* terms. From that point of view, the default position is that everyone should be treated equally, that everyone's rights should be equally respected. Each human life is of equal worth, and so equally deserving of medical care for its preservation. Thus, it is not just to use medical resources to prolong youthful lives but not the lives of those who have already lived a normal span (or, of course, vice versa). Each human being, no matter what their age, has the same worth also in respect of the prevention of pain, distress or disability by medical means. It is no more just to prefer medical attention for alleviating the pain or increasing the mobility of a 20-year-old than for doing the same for an 80-year-old. To divert resources from old people, at the cost of ending their lives more quickly than they would otherwise, and especially of making the last years of anyone's life (except those who have private wealth, or can impose the burden of their care on family members) miserable because uncared for, is to imply that the life of an old person is of less value than that of someone younger. The only result can be a general deterioration in respect for older people, and so a general decline in the moral quality of the society in question.

Part of Callahan's case depends on the premise that the frantic pursuit of technological advance in medicine results in demands being made on medicine which cannot be met without ultimately uncontrollable increases in costs. It is also crucial to what Callahan has to say that these demands are most unjustified when made by older people, because they result from a wish to defy nature, in the sense of rejecting the traditional view of old age as a period of quiet serenity and wisdom before death, in which part of the wisdom is simply to accept one's frailty rather than demand medical help to overcome it. This is why he thinks that the crisis of medicine is in a very special sense a crisis of ageing, needing to be solved by scaling down the demands of old people on the medical system. As a sociological picture of modern Western culture, there are certainly elements of truth in this. People do increasingly look to medicine, not only for relief of pain and prevention of premature death, but also for enhancement of life. Examples which come to mind are the prescription of Prozac, not simply to relieve the symptoms of clinical depression, but in order to make people feel happier in a more positive sense; or the suggested use of gene therapy, not merely to eliminate distressing and painful hereditary illnesses but to positively enhance a person's looks, or temperament or IQ. It is certainly arguable that we should avoid this tendency to regard the role of medicine as being to promote personal satisfaction in this way, rather than to relieve pain and to save lives.

But several comments need to be made on this. First, this should be easier to do in the NHS, which has often been wrongly criticised as a 'National Illness Service', concentrating on the relief of suffering rather than on 'healthcare' in the broader sense. 'Wrongly' criticised, because the promotion of health is better achieved by socio-economic means – better housing, cleaner environment, higher incomes leading to healthier lifestyles, and so on – whereas medicine is at its most effective when it concentrates on reducing *ill* health by curing or treating diseases. Secondly, many reductions of ill health do have positive consequences for the quality of life, as hip replacements increase the mobility of arthritis sufferers or kidney transplants make life much better for sufferers from renal disease. To have a blanket rejection of technological medicine of the kind which Callahan favours would thus be to deny, not only the positive improvements of life which that medicine brings but also its capacity to relieve suffering and disability, which Callahan professes to value in old age as much as in any other phase of life. Thirdly, Callahan can give no reason for seeing this crisis of technological medicine as arising mainly from the excessive demands of *old* people rather than of people in Western society generally. Hence, he is not entitled to say that old people ought to bear the greater responsibility for ending it. In the next chapter, we shall move on from that last point to develop some general conclusions about the alleged crisis.

Chapter 9

A crisis of ageing?

Are old people a burden?

So will there be a crisis of ageing in the NHS? If the discussions of previous chapters show anything, it is that this is far from being a simple question to interpret, let alone to answer. It seems reasonably clear that in most countries more and more people are surviving to older and older ages, and that a declining birth rate means that the rise in the numbers of older people is not being balanced by a parallel increase in the numbers of the young. It is also commonly assumed, and with some basis in empirical evidence, that older people tend to make greater calls on medical services than do those in the prime of life; the fact that, at least in developed countries like the UK, the general health of younger people has improved because of better social conditions and nutrition in earlier life increasingly has postponed ill health to a later age. This is especially true about terminal illnesses: 80% of people in the UK are now aged 65 or more when they die, and the year before death is usually the time of the highest use – and costs – of medical care (although this is less obvious in older than in younger people (*see* Chapter 2). Furthermore, it is undeniably true that the costs of providing a comprehensive health service are continually rising, fuelled by increasingly sophisticated technology which can do much more for patients than was even imaginable when the NHS was founded, and by the inevitably concomitant rise in patient demand for these often expensive treatments. On the other hand, the literature cited in Chapter 2 suggests that there is at least room for doubt whether the costs of caring for an increasing number of older people make any significant contribution to this general rise, and so create anything that could be called a 'crisis'. This is not to deny that there may be a crisis of ever-increasing demands and costs: the issue is the attribution of its cause.

The perception of a crisis as a direct result of ageing depends on seeing an ageing population as a *burden* on society as a whole, and particularly on those members who are of working age and whose taxes provide the bulk of the funding for a system such as the NHS. In imaginative terms, the picture is more or less that painted in the quotation from Andrew Blaikie's book given in Chapter 1 – of a mass of unproductive and unhealthy old people requiring care which drains away the resources created by the labour of a diminished number of younger people and so denies those young people proper satisfaction of their own needs. Expressed in superficially more 'rational' language, it is the prospect described by such writers as Callahan and Battin of a misuse of social resources in a desperate attempt to keep people alive beyond any kind of reasonable lifespan, thus creating an unsustainable situation (Callahan) which is unfair to younger people, on whose care these same resources could be used with much greater benefit (Battin). The perceived crisis, in other words, is not purely financial, it is a crisis of *fairness*, or, as we said in Chapter 4, an *ethical* crisis. The belief is that the ageing of the population challenges the whole moral foundation of such systems as the NHS. However, it can challenge only those systems which are believed to have a moral foundation, and to the extent that they have a moral foundation. A pure market system of medical provision, if such a thing existed, would face no ethical crisis. The US system faces one only to the extent that it is not a pure market system, but includes elements of a moral character. But the ethical crisis, if there is to be one, will be most acute for those systems whose ideological basis is that they serve a moral purpose, of guaranteeing what is held to be a universal human right of access to medical care and of expressing a sense of social solidarity in which all contribute according to their abilities and from which all benefit according to their needs. The systems with which we are most concerned, the NHS in Britain and the Scandinavian systems, are prime examples of what we are talking about.

It may or may not be true that there is a growing resistance to such ideas of solidarity and social justice in Western societies: that those who pay taxes are increasingly reluctant to pay to provide for the needs of others who may not contribute themselves, or who may contribute too little in tax to pay for their own medical needs. For those who share this anti-solidaristic attitude, no doubt the non-contributors (who would include the old, or at least the less affluent among them) are seen as a burden, a drag on the ability of the taxpayers to pursue their own aims, using their own resources. If this were a matter of sociological fact, then it would certainly be more and more unwelcome, given an ageing population, to sustain the NHS in its present form. But the question that concerns us here is one about the *interpretation* of this alleged sociological fact. Is the perception of the old as a burden a mere expression of selfishness, and a rather short-sighted selfishness at that, since all of those who are now young and healthy will, if they are lucky, one day be old themselves and quite possibly frail and in need of medical care? Or is it a perception of a genuine *injustice* done to the young and healthy by the need to provide for those who are old and frail? Only if the latter interpretation is correct is there a crisis facing the moral foundation of the NHS and one that is attributable to an ageing population.

To decide whether the perception of old people as a burden in this second sense is justified we need, as we have done in this work, to examine a number of other questions.

- What, for instance, are the genuine medical *needs*, and so the rights, of older people? To settle this has required us to think about the proper place of old age in the general pattern of a satisfactory human life.
- To what extent can we see access to the kinds of provision made possible by modern high-technology medicine as included in the right to medical care?
- Would it be unfair to older people to restrict (or even deny altogether) their access to such provision, or unfair to younger people *not* to limit the old in this way?

These are very fundamental questions about the nature of the right to medical care and its relation to the purposes of medicine, and they require open acknowledgement and debate.

Is age relevant?

If the moral right to medical care depends on the contribution that medicine can make to an acceptable life for a human being, one which is worthy of human dignity, then we have to ask what that contribution is. It is clear that at least part of it is to relieve pain, distress and disability and to prevent premature death. These might be regarded as, in themselves, negative benefits, but their consequences are normally positive. For someone who has been in pain to live a life free from pain is a positive good; to be delivered from disability is to become able to do things which were previously impossible; to be saved from death is to have the positive benefit of more years (or months, weeks or days) of life; and so on. What is not so clear is whether it is, or ought to be, any part of the purpose of medicine to bring about positive wellbeing *directly* – to enhance the quality of life above the normal. Medicine can make us well in the sense of being free from illness or disability, but should it make us healthy in some more positive way? Many might argue that that is something that ought not to, indeed, cannot, be achieved by medical technology, but by personal effort on the part of the individual who wishes to be fit in this way – by exercise, proper diet, and similar means; and that if someone cannot achieve enhancement by these methods the proper response is not to seek medical help but simply to accept one's limitations. To give medicine the role of trying to enhance nature in this way is in effect to treat the natural human condition as an illness, to medicalise normal human unhappiness or physical imperfection. Certainly, it cannot be argued that, in a system of publicly-funded medicine like the NHS, there is a duty on the state to improve people's lives by medical means in this way (although there may be a duty on the state, outside medical care, to provide the social and economic conditions in which people have a better chance of improving their own lives).

There is a problem here, however: one which sounds like a purely intellectual worry, but which in fact has important practical implications, some of them relevant to our overall theme. One consequence of the development of medical technology is that many sources of human distress which had previously seemed unchangeable parts of the natural order, and so simply to be endured, have become capable of removal or alleviation by medical means. Such examples include various forms of infertility which can at least be bypassed by IVF or artificial insemination. The debates about these cases have already begun. Should we treat infertility as an illness, and IVF as a treatment to which we have a right on the NHS, even if it is highly expensive? Or should we regard it rather, as it was traditionally in the West, as a misfortune, which those afflicted must find some way of coping with? There is a parallel here to ageing, also traditionally seen as a misfortune that we must simply accept and put up with as best we can. Some may be lucky enough to grow older without ageing in the sense of becoming frailer and less active; others may be able to postpone the worst effects of ageing by good living conditions, good diet and plenty of physical and mental exercise. But, on the traditional view, there was little or nothing that medicine as such could do to prevent ageing and its effects. Part of the 'modernised' view of ageing of which Callahan speaks, however, is that improved medical technology is increasingly able to stave off, and may ultimately be able (perhaps through genetic manipulation) to prevent altogether, the least desired effects of growing old. Should we therefore regard access to such medical treatments as part of our right to medical care? Or should we rather, as Callahan thinks, revert to a more traditional view and learn to put up with the frailties of old age, which are he thinks compensated for in part by the advantages of wisdom and experience which also accrue to those who have lived longer?

Part of the reason for Callahan's preference for this more traditional view seems to be aesthetic – that it is more dignified to grow old gracefully than to pretend to be younger than one is (especially if the rejuvenation has to be achieved by medical means). But this is more subjective than most aesthetic evaluations. There seems no rational reason why it is more dignified for an old person to need a wheelchair or a Zimmer frame to get about than to have hip or knee surgery which would enable her to walk naturally. An old person surely has as much right to medical treatment which will provide reasonable mobility as anyone of any other age. Similarly, however admirable stoic resignation to the prospect of death may be at any age, this does not seem to constitute a reason for denying to older patients, but not to younger patients, the right to medical treatment which would make death less imminent. As was argued earlier, the *number* of years added may well be no greater in the case of a young person than in that of an old, and is anyway irrelevant from the moral point of view: the right to life is a basic human right, whose existence implies that one is entitled to medical treatment which has a reasonable chance of preventing death and so prolonging life, no matter whether it is for one year or for 50 years.

Callahan's main argument against the modernised view of ageing, as we have seen, is that it creates uncontrollable costs for the medical care system. Our essential counter-arguments to Callahan's position have already been stated in the previous chapter, but they can be restated here in somewhat different terms, by way of arriving at some general conclusions about the alleged crisis of ageing. Any publicly-funded system must, of course, seek to use resources responsibly, which means, among other things, containing costs as far as is possible while still meeting the central purposes of the system. The responsibility to control costs is itself a moral duty. It is unfair to those who have contributed the resources (the taxpayers, in the case of the NHS) to use them extravagantly. Equally, however, it is unfair to them to fail to use the resources they have contributed to achieve the purposes for which they have established the system. In the case of the NHS, as we have argued, that purpose is primarily to express a sense of social solidarity, by providing medical care for those in most need of it. To contain costs in a way which defeated that object would be as unjust to those who contributed the resources as to fail to control costs at all. This is true *regardless* of whose needs it may be which are chiefly responsible for the rise in costs, that is, even if the rise in the numbers of old people is the primary cause for the upward spiral in the costs of medical care, it does not follow that it would be just to control costs by failing to meet the genuine medical needs of old people, while not making similar savings in the care of younger people. This is even more obviously the case if, as has been shown in Chapter 2, the principal cause for rising medical costs is not the ageing of the population, but the increased demand by *all* age groups for more medical care including expensive high-technology medicine. If there is an impending crisis for medical care, it would be better to describe it as a crisis of modern medicine, affecting the old no more than the young.

To meet this crisis, costs must certainly be controlled, but in a way consistent with the purposes of the system. How can that be done? The only way that seems to meet the demands of solidarity is to introduce some system of rationing in accordance with moral principles, that is, that resources should be allocated in accordance with need. Those in greatest need should have the first call on the use of resources, and others should be ranked in accordance with their degree of need. We have argued that there is no basis for regarding the medical needs of older people as either less or more important than those of younger people, so that there is no justification for treating age in years as a criterion to be used in any such rationing scheme. It is true, as a matter of fact, that older people tend to have greater medical needs than younger people, but it is also true that this is only a tendency, not a necessary connection; old people are individuals who differ very much among themselves, in degree of vulnerability as much as in any other respect. Their medical needs are thus, as much as with younger people, an *individual* matter, not a feature of their age as such, so that there is no reason here for using age as a rationing criterion.

Talk about 'rationing on the basis of medical need', it may reasonably be objected, is far too vague to be of much use for the practical purposes of formulating NHS policy or making clinical decisions. To make it less vague, and more practically useful, we need to be much clearer about what counts as a 'medical need', and in particular which medical needs ought to be satisfied as of right. One of the ways in which it is accurate to speak of a 'crisis of modern medicine' is that the increased possibilities for what can be done for patients as a result of the developments in medical technology force us to think harder about which of these 'things that can be done' constitute genuine medical *needs*. To count as a need, it seems that it must meet two conditions:

- it must be a genuine, objective *benefit* to the patient
- it must be something that can be achieved only by medical treatment of some kind.

For a medical need to count as the basis of a human right to medical care of the relevant kind, it must be something the satisfaction of which is necessary to a life worthy of a human being, so that society is obliged to ensure that the human being in question has access to the means of satisfying it. And any system of rationing that is to be considered *just* or *fair* must clearly be one which secures to all relevant people all medical needs which count as rights in this way.

The problem which arises in a modern multicultural society, in which there is little general consensus about what is 'a life worthy of a human being', and therefore what the conditions for achieving such a life might be, is to arrive at an agreement among all those affected about which medical needs should be regarded as rights. In practice, prioritisation does take place in the NHS, but it often seems to be the outcome, not of applying any rational, let alone any moral, principle, but of the triumph of those who can assert most pressure. Those groups of patients who lose out as a result of such decisions taken within the care system naturally, and to some extent justifiably, see all euphemistically-called prioritisation of medical care as driven simply by the desire for cost-containment, to save the taxpayer at the expense of avoidable suffering for the sick. It seems clear, however, as Daniels and Sabin argue in their articles cited in Chapter 6 (Daniels and Sabin, 1997; Sabin and Daniels, 2002), that allocation decisions in any medical system, especially one which is publicly funded, should not only be transparent but should be arrived at by a process of public consultation. But how can this be possible in as diverse a society as those of the UK and other industrialised countries? Several countries or states have tried, notably Sweden, New Zealand, The Netherlands and the US state of Oregon. Of these, all have attempted public consultation; Sweden is alone in having set principles for choice rather than specific priority programmes but all have met with difficulty in obtaining agreement to an equitable precise allocation of resources (Hunter, 1997). Hunter quotes a unanimous agreement at a 1995 international conference on choices in healthcare that a guaranteed entitlement to healthcare was impossible to operationalise (*see also* Appendices 2 and 3). In the UK, such agreement has not been attempted; instead, UK policy is to pursue clinical effectiveness as the only grounds for choosing which forms of treatment to provide (Hunter, 1997).

Perhaps we should not be too pessimistic, however. At least some, admittedly *very* general, principles would be accepted by most people in societies with state medical care, no matter what differences there might be in their more detailed values. They would be agreed because they seem to follow fairly directly from the basic purpose for having a publicly-funded medical system at all. Human beings have developed medicine as a body of knowledge and skills that enables them to avoid, or at least alleviate, some of the ills that flesh is heir to, notably:

- unnecessary pain
- distress and disability
- premature death.

Because we are members of a society, with a moral obligation to do what we can to reduce each other's misfortunes, we have set up a 'solidaristic' medical care system to ensure that all members of society, no matter what their financial position, can have access to the medical means to avoid these ills. Although this is very general, if we can follow it through we can perhaps gain some insight into the outline of what might be involved in a fair system of rationing of medical care, and one which would be generally acceptable even in a multicultural society. We can also in the process reinforce the earlier point about the irrelevance of age as such to medical rights.

By these criteria, it seems fairly clear that the relief of pain is a medical need, and that pain-relieving treatment ought to be available to all as a matter of right. It seems equally obvious that the more severe the pain the greater the need for, and the right to, pain relief. Furthermore, since the pain of old people is no less severe than that of young people, and since the pain suffered by young people is no more likely to be 'unnecessary' than that suffered by old people, it follows that age has no relevance to the right to pain-relieving treatment. Much the same could be said about the relief of disability. To be unable to move freely, or to see, or hear, etc. may be as distressing for old people as for young. Callahan, and those who think like him, might of course argue that, on a more traditional view of ageing, such disabilities would simply be accepted as part of the natural process of decline, and so would not be so distressing. But the traditional way of thinking also encouraged greater stoicism about disability and pain among people of *all* ages, for the very simple reason that there was little or nothing which medicine could do to improve things. There seems no morally acceptable reason for saying that younger people should enjoy the benefits of medical progress in these ways while denying them to those who are older. If so, there is a strong argument for saying that older people should have precisely the same right to treatment for disability as people of any other age. To be fair to him, Callahan would probably accept at least some treatment for disabilities for old people but would, in line with his desire to control medical costs, oppose any treatment that could be described as 'enhancement' – designed to improve the quality of life beyond the level which would be normal for older people. The problem then would be how to draw the line between 'enhancement' and relief of disability. Hip replacements, to use a stock example, certainly relieve a disability, but also raise the quality of life above what was traditionally thought normal for older people. Hip replacements are relatively economical, but similar arguments might be used about more expensive treatments like organ transplantation, bypass surgery and so on. If these are to be rationed on the grounds of cost, then there does not seem to be any moral argument for applying that rationing to older patients only, rather than to the population as a whole. (Denying this kind of treatment to patients on the grounds of insufficient benefit *might* as it happens be more often relevant to older patients, but that is not a reason for denying it to *all* older people simply because they are old.)

The right to life is widely regarded as the most fundamental human right of all, and is often connected with the medical duty to save lives. But there are tangled moral questions here. The right to life is essentially the right not to be killed, not to have one's life taken away from one by violent and intentional action on the part of another human being. Its relevance to medicine is that it is the basis of the argument against medical euthanasia. But the medical duty to save lives is logically distinct from the medical duty not to kill: it is the duty to use medical means to prevent someone dying prematurely from natural causes (disease or injury). It has been a long-standing tradition in Western moral and theological thought that we can draw a distinction in this context between 'ordinary' and 'extraordinary' means of preventing death. In this tradition, it is a duty laid upon doctors to use all *ordinary* means to prevent death, but there is no duty on any doctor to use *extraordinary* means. Roughly speaking, what this means is that there is no duty to go to great lengths to save a life, if that life will not really be of any benefit to the person in question (e.g. if she will live only for a very short time, or be unconscious for the remainder of her life, or in unbearable pain or distress). Now, the question of the benefit of continued life, while it can arise for patients of any age, is particularly liable to arise, increasingly nowadays, in the case of patients who are older, and so nearer the natural end of their life anyway. But it does not follow that anyone forfeits the right to (even expensive) life-prolonging treatment simply on the grounds of their advanced age. Given the obvious fact that both older and younger people are individuals with different capacities to benefit from treatment, each case must still be judged on its merits, in terms of the individual's need, rather than on the basis of the age of the patient. If it is still true, as Aaron and Schwartz (1984) reported, that there is covert age-based rationing in the NHS of such life-saving treatments as kidney dialysis, concealed by the false claim that older patients (just by virtue of being old) will not necessarily benefit from the treatment, then this is unethical on at least two grounds because:

- it is denying older patients what is as much their right as it is that of younger people
- it is telling lies in order to conceal this denial of rights.

Finally, we must consider a different type of human right, which is often ignored in discussions about rationing because its relevance to the allocation of resources is not so obvious. This is the right to preserve one's autonomy, in the sense of retaining as much as possible of one's control over one's own life. In liberal Western culture, it is regarded as an essential component of human dignity that one should have such autonomy, and therefore the right to respect for autonomy is taken to be fundamental, in ethics in general and in medical ethics in particular. As a human right, it must apply to all human beings, regardless of such differences as age. But does it have resource implications? It can for older people, as for any who are liable to be more vulnerable and so to be more dependent on others. This point emerged very strongly in our discussions in the Centre for Philosophy, Technology and Society (CPTS) research group, especially from the contributions of our colleague Vilhjalmur Arnason, reporting on the Icelandic experience (*see* Appendix 3). Two examples may illustrate it.

1   To secure conditions in such institutions as care homes and geriatric wards which will support patient autonomy, in the face of all the pressures towards a more paternalistic mode of care, may require such forms of provision as individual rooms, in which patients can bring at least some of the familiar items from their own homes which help them to retain a sense of their own identity and worth: these forms of provision obviously carry a cost.
2   Maintaining autonomy in old age may well require that old people should stay in their own homes for as long as possible, but their ability to do this will often mean that help with home cleaning, shopping, cooking of meals and other basic functions is needed, all of which of course requires to be paid for.

It could be argued that preservation of autonomy is a greater need in the case of old people than much medical care of the more traditional kind and that, if anything, greater resources should be allocated to it, within the overall budget for the care of older people, than to straight medical treatment.

It is not our aim in this book to offer detailed policy proposals, but only to clarify the ethical issues involved in making policy about the care of older people and the use of NHS resources. Nevertheless, it may be useful in conclusion to summarise briefly some of the main themes that have emerged in the course of our analysis of the idea of an 'impending crisis of ageing'. It is understandable that, because there are now more people surviving to old age and they are the main users of both hospital services and long-term care, the sense of a resource crisis for the caring services is attributed to the fact of an ageing population. This, however, is much too simplistic. Both the empirical evidence we have examined, and the moral and philosophical arguments we have considered, suggest first of all that it is simply misleading, and clouds the ethical issues, to talk of a 'crisis of *ageing*' at all. Empirically, it is questionable whether or to what extent any sharp rise in the costs of the medical care system is due to the ageing of the population. Certainly other factors, such as the increased use of and demand for expensive high-technology medicine in diagnosis and treatment at all ages, seem to play a significant part. Morally speaking, we have argued that, even if the demands on the system made by an ageing population *do* play a major part in the rise in costs, it by no means follows that the costs ought to be controlled by cutting back on the medical provision for older people and concentrating resources on the care of the young. Nor is it relevant, as we have tried to show, that it is the young and employed who provide the bulk of those resources through their taxes. They provide those resources, not in order to meet only their own needs but in a spirit of solidarity, in which those who are best able to do so provide care for those who are most in need of it (whether or not they are the same as the providers). An injustice would be done by satisfying the rights of one group of people while denying satisfaction to another. If costs need to be contained, therefore, it ought to be by a system of rationing which applies to all equally; in effect, which provides most for those who are most in need and least for the least needy.

Furthermore, we may well agree with Callahan that in the modern world we expect too much from medicine and that it would be better to reduce our expectations, but the logic of that position is that we should *all* reduce our demands, not just that the old should. It may also be true that, in an increasingly individualist and market-orientated society, the better off have come to feel resentment at funding the care of others, and that the sense of social solidarity has thereby been weakened. What is important, however, is that people should be aware of the moral cost of abandoning solidarity. To see old people as a burden is to exclude them from the circle of people about whom we should care. In a sense, it is to diminish their humanity. That is both morally undesirable, like treating any other group of human beings as less than fully human, and short-sighted, for the reasons stated earlier. An ethically sustainable publicly-funded medical system, like the NHS, must treat older patients as having the same rights as younger patients, both in clinical decision making and in the formulation of public policy. This is the sense in which the idea of a 'crisis of ageing' distorts moral perceptions.

Chapter 10

Policy implications

So, what can the NHS learn from the philosophical analysis presented here? The context of the analysis was the NHS, and the question was about the impact of ageing on acute care and the implications of any impact. The project set out to:

- decide whether the NHS is facing a crisis as a result of the ageing of the population
- examine the ethical dimensions of proposed and potential responses to this crisis.

The ethical dimensions are the arguments used in support of particular views, i.e. the moral principles (e.g. justice, rights, duty of care, respect for human dignity) that may be explicit or implied. The conclusions were as follows:

1   Despite the growing numbers and proportions of older people in all the countries of the Western world, the crisis-generating increase in demands on the NHS cannot be solely or even directly attributed to this (except to the extent that terminal illness occurs very largely at older ages). However, other sources of tension, especially the potential of new technology and the growing emphasis on the importance of youth, may have a bearing on the care of older people and make them part of the solution to the crisis.
2   An ethical society may be defined as one in which there is general acceptance of certain rules and standards governing how we should relate to each other. The ethical basis of the NHS is justice or fairness to all citizens and there is no moral justification for planning to give less medical care to people solely because they are older: all citizens have equal rights. However, there may be grounds for differential consumption of and access to medical care by different age groups because of what that age implies, and not just because they have different medical conditions. The real question is not absolute but relative. Given the fact that NHS resources are limited, what is the ethical basis for deciding who does get care compared to who does not? Justice does not require strict, mathematical equality of treatment; but what it does require is that deviations from strict equality must be justified by being shown to arise from *morally relevant* differences between people.
3   The gap between supply and demand for the NHS is extremely unlikely to be met solely by attempts to improve its effectiveness and cost-effectiveness. It is not unethical to ration medical care but, because the NHS is a solidaristic system funded very largely from taxation, there is an ethical requirement for openness and participation in deciding who or what should take priority.

Let us now look at current practice in and around the NHS to see how, from an ethical perspective, it fares in respect of these ethical issues.

Criteria for prioritising access to medical care

The government has delineated equality of access to the NHS as meaning access based on need regardless of age, sex, race, creed, geography or ability to pay. Since the mid-1970s, when the rise in oil prices brought home the reality of the costs of public provision, it has acknowledged the need for the NHS to set priorities for the use of resources and has identified medical need and the effectiveness of interventions as the main parameters by which priorities may be chosen. These are common principles across European countries (*see* Appendix 3) and can be accepted as morally relevant potential differences between people and between treatments. In the past decade, through the National Institute for Clinical Excellence (NICE), it has promoted the use of evidence-based guidelines for clinical practice as a means of reducing inequalities in treatments and of ineffective (and therefore inefficient) forms of care. NICE also assesses therapeutic developments and selects which to recommend (or not to recommend) to the NHS on the basis of their cost-effectiveness as judged by quality-adjusted life years (QALYs) gained or, failing that, simply by life years gained (Rawlins and Culyer, 2004). This approach also can be accepted as an ethical way to increase the effectiveness, and cost-effectiveness, of what the NHS has on offer. However, both activities have the effect of pre-empting resources because they promote new forms of care without identifying what services will be withdrawn or which potential consumers will not receive treatment. In this respect the current position is unethical because it creates unknown and unacknowledged inequities in access to acute care (Maynard *et al.*, 2004).

Operationalising the criteria

So, the principles set out by the government are ethically acceptable. Unfortunately, operationalising these principles has been the sticking point for virtually every state in the world that has tried it, either because it is too uncomfortable for individuals and states to name the losers or because the definitions and measurement of need and effectiveness are less than clear or agreed (New, 1998). Until now in the UK, government policy has been to delegate to devolved governments and to local health authorities the management of their existing resources in the face of pre-emptions such as the above, as well as the mandatory improvement of terms and conditions of employment of NHS staff. However, explicit local policies about who or what not to treat are extremely rare – and, indeed, most that have been reported concern upper age limits for access to such high-technology care as renal dialysis and coronary care. In practice, it is left to clinicians to decide how best to use the scarce resources of time, skills and technology that are available to their team. The bases of their judgements are indeed the principles of 'need' and 'effectiveness' but, in the absence of usable definitions, it is the interpretations of these two concepts that vary. At its simplest, 'need' may contain values about urgency, degree of threat to life, patients' wishes and expectations, and the existence of alternative forms of intervention or support; while effectiveness depends at least on the goals of the doctor, the patient and the system that are incorporated in the information from evidence-based studies as well as at the particular consultation. Both parties are highly influenced by experience, both personal and professional, and that includes context (e.g. Abelson, 2001; Eraker and Politser, 1994; Frith, 1999; Light and Hughes, 2002; Butler, 1999).

As a result, there is plenty of evidence that older people receive less acute medical care (Austin and Russell, 2003; Bowling, 1999). What is important from an ethical perspective is that this should not be judged to be discriminatory or ageist unless there is evidence that there are no other grounds, such as clinical effectiveness, from which this effect arises. Such a conclusion is extremely difficult to reach, especially if, for example, the decision not to treat an older person aggressively stems from that person's belief that they have had 'a good life' already, but that is an implicit component of a doctor–patient consultation. There is some evidence that this and related beliefs, which are relics of Calvinism in the post-Calvinist era, are still alive and well in at least parts of the UK (Williams, 1990). Moreover, a proportion of the public would support giving priority to younger people (Kneeshaw, 1997) but, at a policy level, would limit this to when the younger people were more likely to benefit and not because of people's social roles or because the older people were likely to have had more chance to experience life (NICE Citizens' Council, 2004).

They and other consumers would also favour leaving such choices to clinicians on the basis that doctors and nurses are more likely to take the individual's needs and wishes into account. However, it creates increasing tension and guilt for clinicians when they recognise the nature of the comparisons and judgements about individuals that they are being forced to make, and which may conflict with their professional ethic (Butler, 1999). It is also likely to be inequitable across the UK, because each clinician operates in different resource contexts and has many other influences on his or her judgements about what is more worth doing than something else. Given that professional ethics are especially crucial for the protection of the best interests of patients in a non-market healthcare system such as in the UK, this is a responsibility which, arguably, is itself unethical.

Is solidarity still viable?

One of the prevalent misconceptions in the UK about solidarity is the belief that older people deserve to be cared for because of all the taxes and National Insurance that they have paid in the past. This has been quoted by both old and young (NICE Citizens' Council, 2004). However, ethically, there is no right to earmark personal contributions in a solidaristic system; indeed, it is contrary to the very principle of solidarity and the ethical requirement for a 'veil of ignorance', at the time of contributing, about what the future may hold for you or anyone else. (Arguably there is a difference between the UK, one of the few countries in which 83% of the healthcare system is funded from general taxation, and other European countries, in which most of the public funding comes from social insurance, which might be expected to be based in part on individual risk.) If solidarity is to be upheld, it is important for citizens to understand this, as it may affect attitudes to the 'just deserts' of older people.

A major concern in all industrialised countries with state provision of medical care is the influence of the late twentieth century's individualistic ethos on the survival of solidarity as the basis for medical care provision (*see* Appendix 2). Ashcroft *et al.* (2000) have described, from a philosophical perspective, the historical tension between classical liberalism and what they call 'statism' (where the state was considered morally responsible for the wellbeing and safety of its subjects); and the importance of the 'Third Way' to the concept of solidarity. They argue that it replaces the economic underpinning of socialism with a focus on the importance of social factors and social inclusion. These require a new look at 'what a state is actually for'. The answer includes, *inter alia*:

- allowing for both market and civil society but jointly governed by principles of solidarity and social justice
- allowing for responsibilities as a necessary concomitant of rights
- allowing for a 'diverse but egalitarian' society.

But solidarity does not permit indifference.

(On old age specifically, Ashcroft *et al.* (2000) observe that some people attribute the inequality experienced by older people to the Welfare State itself and the creation of dependency and poverty (*see* Appendix 2). One of these is Giddens (1994), one of the founders of the 'Third Way' in politics, whom they quote: 'the welfare system defines old age not as a status worthy of respect but as a disqualification from full membership'. They note also that the principles of the Third Way do not appear to have been actuated in England and Wales (but have been in Scotland) as exemplified by the government's response to the Royal Commission on Long-Term Care. It remains to be seen whether the costs in Scotland will be acceptable when the trade-offs become explicit, or whether public pressure will push England and Wales into matching Scotland's principles.)

One of the main points of their analysis is that, to be ethical, solidarity requires the specification of roles, whereas principles such as justice do not. Houtepen and Ter Meulen (2000b) note the term 'reflective solidarity' introduced by Dean (1995) to describe the combination of solidarity with a 'positive approach to differences'. Thus the conclusion on solidarity is that there is no ethical difficulty in modifying traditional solidaristic medical care with a mixed system that may include some private payment and some social insurance. The point yet again is the need for this to be agreed with the citizens who are the responsibility of the system.

Obtaining citizens' views

This is not the place to rehearse the many reviews that have concluded that consultation and information exchange with the public and patients is the crucial missing factor in the government's current approach to the NHS and, in this context, to priority setting (e.g. Butler, 1999; Coulter and Ham, 2000; Houtepen and Ter Meulen, 2000a; New, 1998; RCPL, 1995). We simply add a philosophical perspective to the debates by agreeing that the current position is unethical. The issue, once more, is how it might be effectively and usefully changed. Although it is recognised as extremely difficult to obtain any kind of representative views on priorities (Hunter, 1997), there is a growing body of recommendations on how it might be done (New, 1998), and some examples of evolving good practice in the UK such as NICE's Citizens' Council, and consultations by the Human Fertilisation and Embryology Authority. INVOLVE, an organisation that promotes the involvement of consumers in health research, has produced guidance for new researchers that is very apposite for public involvement at organisational levels

(INVOLVE, 2004). Almost certainly, there is no single best method, and almost certainly it requires qualitative and quantitative methods in different mixes for different levels, settings and questions. But, we repeat, the current absence of formal governmental attempts to seek representative, non-partisan and partisan, public input to their selection of priorities is unethical. And, of course, such consultation requires the provision of the kind of information about making choices that has been so singularly absent from the management of the NHS. The project therefore concluded that solidarity in respect of medical care in the UK can survive, and, ethically, should accommodate modern individualistic and participative values. However, it requires that the means of incorporating citizens' views be agreed by government and citizens. This means that government and citizens have to share and agree facts about the existing position so that the interpretation of fairness or justice, or even simply the process for deciding what is fair, is visible to all.

NHS principles and priorities 1942–2003

David Austin

In the UK there is a National Health Service, which operates in all four component countries but with some differences of structure and, since devolution of NHS in Scotland policy to the Scottish Parliament in 1997, a few differences of principle. Several themes that are relevant to the care of older people have changed quite markedly since its inception in 1948, and they will be examined in turn:

1 Changing principles and how definitions of important words have changed (mainly 1942–1979).
2 Recognition of financial constraints and the introduction of priorities (since 1976).
3 The relationship between the NHS and social services (since the 1970s).

(*Note*: Although the developments of policy, the exposition of principles and the structure of the NHS have been broadly similar in the four countries of the UK, governmental documents have shown variation in timing and explicitness of statements on principles and priorities especially between Scotland and England/ Wales. What follows is not a comprehensive listing of all government statements or NHS Acts but, rather, a summary of the main trends mainly from the English Department of Health unless there is a relevant variant from elsewhere, usually the Scottish Health Department in Edinburgh. Quotations are in italics.)

NHS statements of principle

The Beveridge Report *Social Insurance and Allied Services*. Report by Sir William Beveridge. (Reprinted 1966, originally 1942.) Cmnd. 6404. Parliament, HMSO, London.

Beveridge, in his wartime report, identified five giants that would require tackling as part of a comprehensive policy of social progress. He identified these as:

- Want
- Disease
- Ignorance
- Squalor
- Idleness.

His proposals on the social security system were to be seen as tackling Want:

> *Scope of Social Security: The term 'social security' is used here to denote the securing of an income to take the place of earnings when they are interrupted by unemployment, sickness or accident, to provide for retirement through age,*

to provide against loss of support by the death of another person and to meet exceptional expenditures, such as connected with birth, death and marriage (para. 300).

He thought that no scheme providing social security would be satisfactory unless certain assumptions were made. The second assumption is quoted below:

Comprehensive health and rehabilitation services for prevention and cure of disease and restoration of capacity to work, available to all members of the community (para. 426).

Although not the point of the report, Beveridge went on to elaborate. He considered it logical in a system that provides sickness and disability benefit to have a complementary health service to ensure that the invalid rapidly returns to work (and therefore off benefit). He also outlined the healthcare that the service would provide:

. . . a comprehensive National Health Service will ensure that for every citizen there is available whatever medical treatment he requires, in whatever form he requires it, domiciliary or institutional, general, specialist or consultant and will ensure the provision also of dental, ophthalmic and surgical appliances, nursing and midwifery and rehabilitation after accidents (para. 427).

. . . the service itself should . . . be provided where needed without contribution conditions in any individual case (para. 427).

A National Health Service (1944) Cmnd. 6502. Ministry of Health and Department of Health for Scotland, HMSO, London.

The White paper lays out in detail the structure and function of the NHS. In the first paragraph it states:

. . . in the future every man, woman and child can rely on getting all the advice and treatment and care which they may need in matters of personal health; that what they get shall be the best medical and other facilities available; that their getting these shall not depend on whether they can pay for them, or on any other factor irrelevant to the real need – the real need being to bring the country's full resources to bear upon reducing ill-health and promoting good health in all its citizens (p. 5).

The White paper also points out that in Scotland there may be differences in organisation but not *of scope or of object*. The *Comprehensive Service for All* was defined in two ways:

- it was available to all
- it covered all necessary forms of healthcare.

The service was to include home care, as well as hospital care, and treat minor ailments, major disease and disabilities. The document included nursing care as an integral part of this free service. On the subject of access to specialist care, the paper states that:

. . . when the need arises . . . everyone can get access . . . to more specialised branches of medicine or surgery (para. 6).

Priority was mentioned in relation to dental care, where attention was to be focused on children, young people, expectant and nursing mothers. This was seen as only a temporary measure, due to the relative shortage of dentists. The explicit aim was, however, to provide a full dental service to the whole population.

Possible charges for certain appliances were mentioned briefly, however the overall tone was undeniably giving people the *right to look to a public service for all their medical needs* [emphasis added].

The proposals were summarised as follows.

> *Objects in view:*
> 1 *To ensure that everybody in the country – irrespective of means, age, sex, or occupation – shall have equal opportunity to benefit from the best and most up-to-date medical and allied services available.*
> 2 *To provide, therefore, for all who want it, a comprehensive service covering every branch of medical and allied activity, from the care of minor ailments to major medicine and surgery; to include the care of mental as well as physical health, and all specialist services; . . . to include all normal general services; . . . and to include all necessary drugs and medicines and a wide range of appliances.*
> 3 *To divorce the care of health from questions of personal means or other factors irrelevant to it; . . .* (p. 47).

The principles subsequently set out were concerned with clinical freedom, patient choice and family doctor service.

Between 1948 and the 1970s there was little or no explicit discussion of Health Service principles. There were NHS Acts in 1949, 1951, 1952, 1957 and 1961, and Hospital Plans for the component countries in 1961 and 1962, but these did not seem to be preceded by any statement of policy. Rather, they were to do with administrative and financial matters such as the introduction of some charges for appliances, as had been foreshadowed in the Beveridge Report.

Health and Welfare: the development of community care (England and Wales) (1963) Cmnd. 1973. Parliament, HMSO, London.

This was complementary to the England and Wales Hospital Plan of 1962. It is significant because it states the needs of four broad groups of people (mothers and young children, the elderly, the mentally disordered, the physically handicapped) in relation to care in the community and preventive medicine. Priorities were not stated but the four main groups that require community care were outlined.

National Health Service: the future structure of the NHS (1970) Department of Health and Social Security, HMSO, London.

This was a Green paper, but the principles of the NHS were restated. It mentioned how the service was financed (through general taxation) and that the NHS should, in principle, be free. The paper conceded that a standardised service was not fully in place in terms of geographical areas, but that much change had occurred since 1948. The clinical freedom of doctors and the 'family doctor' basis of the service were also noted as principles. The document did not use the phrase *Comprehensive Health Service*.

Royal Commission on the National Health Service (1979) Cmnd. 7615. Parliament, HMSO, London.

This report points out that detailed and publicly-declared objectives and principles have not been made regarding the NHS. It suggests that the objectives of the NHS are as follows:

> *We believe the NHS should:*
> *encourage and assist individuals to remain healthy;*
> *provide equality of entitlement to health services;*
> *provide a broad range of services of a high standard;*
> *provide equality of access to these services;*
> *provide a service free at the time of use;*
> *satisfy the reasonable expectations of the users;*
> *remain a national service responsive to local needs* (p. 9).

These objectives, as with the original NHS White paper, should be seen in the context of the time (*see later*). The tone of these objectives seems altogether more guarded than previous statements. It seems as though a *broad range of services* has replaced a *comprehensive service*. *Equality of entitlement* was not stated before, possibly because services were to be distributed to individuals in need. Equality of entitlement means that people of the same need are equally entitled to healthcare (whether they receive it or not). *Satisfying reasonable expectations* is a statement open to considerable interpretation, allowing the possible withholding of treatment if the expectations of the patient are deemed by someone (government/doctor/hospital, etc.) to be unreasonable. The document undertakes a discussion of these principles, accepting that some of the original objectives are perhaps unattainable.

The Patient's Charter (1991) Department of Health, HMSO, London.

This, first ever, charter for patients gave the purpose of the NHS as:

* *to promote good health*
* *to diagnose and treat those who are ill*
* *to provide healthcare for those with continuing needs.*

It also set out the values of the NHS as:

* *to provide fair entitlement and access to its services*
* *to identify and seek the peoples' needs and wishes*
* *to set out and achieve the highest standards possible*
  - *of care and respect for each person*
  - *of results*
  - *of value for money*
* *to improve standards through research, education, monitoring and review* (p. 12).

In the past decade, government concern with the NHS has been to make it more responsive to patients, more efficient, and to ensure that its performance is more publicly assessed and monitored. Its values and principles for access to care have not overtly changed. These trends were responses to both the consumer movement and to financial constraints and crises, which became hot media topics; they are dealt with in the next section.

Recognition of financial constraints and the introduction of priorities

The last 30 or more years has seen a slow (and sometimes not so slow) move away from the 'ideal' of the Comprehensive Service for All towards priorities, value for money, target setting and efficiency. The optimism exuded by the Beveridge Report and 1944 NHS Act eclipsed serious questions of resource. However, the report proclaimed:

> The importance of securing that suitable hospital treatment is available for every citizen and that recourse to it, at the earliest moment when it becomes desirable, is not delayed by **financial considerations** (para. 433).

Of course, Beveridge meant individual financial considerations although, interestingly, he did express a concern even then that *it is dangerous to be in any way lavish to old age, until adequate provision has been assured for all other vital needs, such as the prevention of disease and the adequate nutrition of the young* (para. 236). However, the state perspective was not picked up, and the NHS White paper elaborated:

> ... *that their getting these* [health services] *shall not depend on whether they can pay for them, or on any other factor irrelevant to the real need – the real need being to bring the country's full resources to bear upon reducing ill-health and promoting good health in all its citizens* (p. 5).

The only point of note regarding finance was that certain appliances were to be charged for, although the monies gained from this were to represent (and still do) only a small part of the overall NHS budget.

It is generally accepted that the recognition of financial constraints on public expenditure followed the raising of oil prices in 1973, which had a universal effect on the use of international borrowing and national governments' spending plans in all sectors. In the UK, the first NHS documents to reflect this appeared in both England (for England and Wales) and Scotland in 1976.

Priorities for the Health and Social Services in England (1976) Department of Health and Social Security, HMSO, London.

This was one of two relevant consultative documents produced from London in 1976. The other, *Prevention and Health: everybody's business*, put the first ever NHS policy emphasis on prevention of disease, and the responsibility that each citizen has to themselves and the wider community. Prevention has always been part of the NHS remit; however after the spending restrictions of the mid-1970s this path was more strongly pursued in the belief that it could answer some of the funding problems by reducing ill health and therefore the demand for treatment.

The 'priorities' document represented the *first time an attempt has been made to establish rational and systematic priorities throughout the health and personal social services*. A full review of all spending was conducted, with particular reference to making savings in general/acute hospital services and administration. Growth rates for different sectors were explicitly set (average 2%), for example:

- *services used mainly by the elderly – hospital geriatric provision, home nursing, residential homes, day care, home helps and meals – increase 3.2% a year*
- *services for the mentally handicapped – hospital provision, local authority residential and day care provision – increase 2.8% a year*
- *services for children and families – increase 1.2% a year*
- *expenditure on maternity services – fall by 1.8% a year* (p. 3).

The report acknowledged the problems facing the acute hospital sector – waiting lists, waiting times, increasing numbers of elderly patients and the need to introduce new technologies – but insisted that any resources should be found from savings within the acute sector.

Priorities in primary care were also set – the development of primary healthcare teams, preventive medicine, family planning, and better value in pharmaceutical costs. Primary care was given objectives to fulfil, which included reducing the demands on acute hospital care and allowing for the increased workload that will result from the increasing elderly population.

In terms of the acute service, the document admits that there *is clear evidence of inadequate provision.* The acute sector's main needs were determined as:

- *to reduce waiting times*
- *to reduce geographical disparity, both between and within regions*
- *to facilitate medical advances and improved patterns of care*
- *to provide for the increased numbers of elderly* [mainly geriatric and mental health]
- *to make further improvements in the rehabilitation services* (para. 4.13).

There was also evidence of target setting on the subject of waiting lists; health authorities were unable to meet the targets set (treating urgent cases within one month and all other cases within a year). Services for the elderly, as mentioned, along with physically and mentally handicapped services, were given priority. These services took the form mainly of home help, geriatric services, home nursing and some hospital services (e.g. spinal unit).

Also for the first time, a list of effective healthcare interventions was included as an Appendix. These priorities were ratified in 1977 in *The Way Forward, Priorities in the Health and Social Services* (DHSS, HMSO, London), and in 1981 by *Care in Action – a handbook of policies and priorities for the health and personal social services in England* (DHSS, HMSO, London).

The Way Ahead – The Health Service in Scotland (Memorandum) 1976 (1976) Scottish Home and Health Department, Edinburgh.

The Scottish equivalent was more explicit about priority setting and stated that *the serious economic situation facing the United Kingdom calls for restrictions in public expenditure for some years to come* (para. 1). This prompted the Secretary of State for Scotland to review health priorities and to suggest six principles which Health Boards, the Common Services Agency and *all those engaged in the Health Service* should make their prime consideration.

1   *The need to operate the services within budgets available which allow for a limited measure of growth.*
2   *The need to promote healthcare in the community through the progressive improvement of primary care services and community health services.*

3 *More positive development of health services for families in areas of multiple deprivation.*

4 *Lessening the growth of the acute sector of the hospital service in order to finance developments in other sectors.*

5 *Continued improvements in hospital and community health services for the elderly, the mentally ill, the mentally handicapped and the physically handicapped.*

6 *Encouragement of preventive measures and the development of a fully responsible attitude to health on the part of the individual and the community* (p. 3).

The document recognised that health authorities would be faced with *difficult decisions over priorities*. The Scottish Office did not attempt to make these *difficult decisions* by imposing a *uniform pattern of development*. Instead, they delegated responsibility onto the local health authorities, which were to arrive at their priorities depending on local circumstances. The document considered the regular increase in funding of the NHS to have *removed the stimulus to make a comprehensive appraisal of priorities across all the various sectors of the NHS*. The need for an *explicit* appraisal of priorities was forced by the economic situation, not by a fundamental rethink of principle. In any event, a list of priority groups was established, to whom more resources would be directed through savings in other sectors and small increases in overall expenditure. The priority groups were:

> . . . *care of the elderly, the mentally ill, the mentally handicapped, and the physically handicapped* . . . (p. 7).

In particular, attention focused away from what it described as the *paradox of the present system that so much is spent on ineffective cure while so little is done to encourage the public in general to improve its own health,* but it did not list specific effective interventions. Services to be *rationalised* were described as *less essential*. The main area for cut backs was the hospital sector where acute and maternity services were considered to be over-provided. Beds and often wards were to be closed where they were considered relatively expensive to run (this would have almost certainly meant restricted access for some people). The government described the possible consequence of service rationalisation:

> . . . *it may not be possible to meet the convenience of some patients without detriment to the health and safety of others* (p. 15).

It is distinctly possible that unequal access to healthcare resulted from these proposals. This differential access may have been geographical (different priorities in different areas) as well as in specific groups of people. The redirection of resources into long-term community and hospital care for the elderly and mental health obviously gave these priority groups greater potential for access in these areas. It is possible to say that anyone outside the priority groups would not be entitled to equal access to healthcare, because of the comparative underfunding in other areas. There is no evidence from this document, however, that any group of people were systematically denied access to a particular treatment (although this is not to say it did not happen); the focus was on the top end (priorities) not the bottom end (which diseases or services might not get care).

The concentration of resources on care of the elderly was because of the projected rise in the number of people over 75 years old. These increased resources were mainly to be concentrated on maintaining independence for the elderly, for example geriatric and long stay services. Hospital services for the elderly were to be subject to constant scrutiny – possibly implying a limitation of access to acute services. As in England, this seminal document was developed and implemented through the SHAPE and SHARPEN reports: *Scottish Health Services Planning Council. Scottish Health Priorities for the Eighties (SHAPE)* (1980) (HMSO, Edinburgh) and *SHARPEN (Scottish Health Authorities Review of Priorities for the Eighties and Nineties)* (1988) (HMSO, Edinburgh).

Health Committee – First Report. Priority setting in the NHS: purchasing (1995) Vol. 1. HMSO, London.

This was the government document that dealt most specifically with the fundamentals of priority setting. It was from a cross-party committee and not government policy; it outlined the reasons why resources had failed to keep up with demand (increasing expectations/demography/technological advances) and examined (and rejected for the UK's purposes) the Oregon formula. (The Oregon formula ranked diagnosis/treatment pairs by different means (in a trial and error fashion) until an agreed list of priorities had been arrived at. The state would then fund down to a certain level, effectively excluding certain treatments. Public meetings were held to get public opinion on wider health issues and to educate them on the formula.)

The report pointed out the general issues raised by this method.

- *Firstly, an objective assessment of service priorities requires a large volume of reliable information on health needs; information on the effectiveness of individual treatments particularly in terms of clinical outcome; and information on service costs. The Oregon approach has highlighted the paucity of such data.*
- *Secondly, the approach has underlined the need to secure effective public involvement in decision making and ultimately public backing for the resultant decisions* (p. vii).

Significantly, the Oregon plan decided that for *reasons of equity, . . . age and lifestyle factors such as smoking could not be used to deny treatment.* Of course, the Oregon plan has to be seen in the context of the US system – this was only looking at rationing Medicare and Medicaid – as opposed to the whole population in the NHS.

On our healthcare system the report said of rationing:

> *Choices are not new. Choices on the use of resources in the NHS are made every day of the week, every week of the year. Traditionally such priorities tended to be more implicit than explicit – 'set by history and stealth' as one witness put it* (p. vii).

The report considered local purchasers to have the responsibility for deciding what was important. This could leave the likelihood of serious discrepancies in what services were provided in different geographical areas – creating inequity and discrepancies in accessibility.

The report also noted the variation in these principles between different agencies, although few were explicit. One health authority (North Essex) worked with the following.

- *Equity – people with comparable needs should receive the same standard of care, regardless of where they live in North Essex or are treated.*

- *Acceptability – healthcare should be provided in a manner that satisfies the reasonable expectations of individuals and the community.*
- *Appropriateness – healthcare should meet the needs of individuals and the population as a whole and be responsive to changing needs.*
- *Effectiveness – healthcare should achieve the intended outcome for the individual.*
- *Efficiency – resources should be used to best effect in obtaining intended outcomes.*
- *Accessibility – those in need should have ready access to health care which should be provided as locally as possible* (p. xiv).

The report considered equity, public choice and effectiveness to be the three main principles. It called for an explicit statement of ethical principles to guide priority setting.

The 1990s saw considerable discussion across the UK about what were the most important principles; in general, the same three as above emerged at local levels. On priority setting, it should be clear from the above that there has never been the slightest hint at government level that older people 'should' have less access to medical care than younger people, although the practical implications of some of the disease priorities may have had that effect. Indeed, they have appeared as a 'top' priority on several occasions.

Since that time, the NHS throughout the UK has continued the use of priorities and targets as a means of allocating and trying to control expenditure but the prime concern of policy has been with the balance and relationships between health and personal social services, which is considered in the next section.

The relationship between the NHS and social services

National Health Service: the future structure of the NHS (1970) Department of Health and Social Security, HMSO, London.

This document (a Green paper) proposed NHS restructuring (unifying the authorities that provided different sectors of care). One of the reasons the paper gave to back up its argument on unification was as follows:

> *When deciding what priority to give their* [local authorities] *health services as against the competing needs of their other services, it is clearly difficult for local authorities to take full account of the advantages which would accrue to the health services as a whole* (p. 4).

The outcome across the UK was the removal of responsibility for disease prevention, health education, personal care and human public health services from local government into a unified NHS (although primary care remained independent contractors) (**1974 NHS Act**). This structure has remained in place, although recent trends have been to enforce better interaction and collaboration between the NHS and local government (*see below*).

Caring for People: community care in the next decade and beyond (1989) Cmnd. 849. Department of Health, HMSO, London.

This White paper along with the Working for Patients document preceded the NHS and Community Care Act 1990. The main purpose was to separate 'health' (or, more strictly, medical care) provided 'free' by the NHS from social care provided by local government (and means-tested) and the voluntary and private sectors. The government gave what it described as the *key components* of community care as:

- *services that respond flexibly and sensitively to the needs of individuals and their carers*
- *services that allow a range of options for consumers*
- *services that intervene no more than necessary to foster independence*
- *services that concentrate on those with the greatest needs* (p. 5).

The role of the social services was outlined as follows:

- *carrying out an appropriate assessment of an individual's need for social care (including residential and nursing home care), in collaboration as necessary with medical, nursing and other caring agencies, before deciding what services should be provided*
- *designing packages of services tailored to meet the assessed needs of individuals and their carers. The appointment of a 'case manager' may facilitate this*
- *securing the delivery of services, not simply by acting as direct providers, but by developing their purchasing and contracting role to become enabling authorities* (p. 17).

The responsibility for nursing home care in the community thus became at the discretion of the social services rather than based on clinical need. As the decision is a *social* rather than a *medical* one, the provision of a means-tested, rather than a free, service became a dilemma. The distinction hung (and still hangs) on the definition of personal care (a social service) and when this becomes nursing care (a medical service). Considerable time and effort has been devoted to this issue since the Act; the two main national reports are summarised below.

Long-term Care Future Provision and Funding: Government response to the third report from the Health Committee (1996) Cm. 3457. HMSO, London.

On the funding of long-term care the government stated their belief that there should *be a balance of responsibility between taxpayers and individuals in meeting the costs*. As noted above, this was a change, in principle, from when long-term care was considered a priority of the NHS. The Health Committee pointed out the injustice of the present system:

> . . . the nursing costs of long-term care should be the responsibility of the NHS . . . [this] would tackle the most manifest unfairness of the present system, the way 'health care' is currently defined to exclude 'nursing care in nursing homes'. . . . It is clearly illogical and indefensible that whereas someone who is ill in a hospital acute ward receives free nursing care, another person with similar medical problems who is cared for in a nursing home is means-tested for their nursing care. . . . 'physical location rather than the individual's needs, determines whether or not the NHS pays for care' (p. 10).

The committee went on to express their view that this represented discrimination on the grounds of age. The government's reply was that *it does not believe that it currently represents the highest priority for extra NHS expenditure*. This is in direct contrast to earlier statements of priority, which put care of the elderly at the top of the list.

The issue of local eligibility creating inequity was also addressed in the report:

> . . . *given the great historic variation in the balance and level of local services it* [the government] *does not consider that it would be feasible to introduce national eligibility criteria at this stage without major service disruption and without undermining local flexibility* (p. 5).

Thus it appears that by 1996 a combination of the above policy on long-term care, target setting in primary care and target setting in acute care, the elderly were being denied access to the NHS at many levels. Not only that, but cost shifting between the NHS and the social services was taking place, excluding most elderly people who needed nursing home care from a free service. Inequitable access to long-term care was therefore created on three levels:

- old versus young
- type of disease and care required
- relative wealth of the individual.

With Respect to Old Age. Report by the Royal Commission into Long-Term Care (1999) Cm. 4192-I. The Stationery Office, London.

The new Labour government elected in 1997 commissioned this report (called the Sutherland Report) following an Audit Commission review of long-term care expenditure (Sutherland, 1999). Its aim was 'to find a sustainable system of funding of long-term care for elderly people, both in their own homes and in other settings'. It noted that:

> . . . [the NHS] *appears to be increasingly driven by performance measures which encourage it to treat people and get them out of hospital as quick as possible – perhaps too quickly in the case of older people* (1.5).

A possible reason for restructuring funding and services, therefore, was to allow local authorities to determine their priorities from the best possible position. This was meant in the context of providing the proper care by stopping the motivation for cost shifting. This practice involved keeping patients who could be discharged in hospital (paid for by the hospital service) to prevent the cost of community care (paid for by the local authority).

The commission was scathing about the inherent inequity in the current system of providing long-term care. It made the point about individuals with different diseases having unequal access to free treatment, and also pointed out the trend in the NHS towards concentrating on acute medical care and neglecting long-term care (38% decrease of long-stay beds since 1983 and an increase of 900% in private nursing) – contrary to the priorities set out during the 1980s. However, it recognised, as did Beveridge, the shared responsibility between the individual and the state, and the need to share risk. Its conclusions, which are very relevant to this study, highlighted the need for a change in intergenerational interactions and presented a new, very positive attitude to old age. The values of the commission were a positive view of ageing:

- as a valuable part of society
- as a natural part of life not a burden
- as an opportunity for intellectual fulfilment and achievement of other ambitions

- it should not be compartmentalised
- long-term care should be a set of positive actions not a management of decline
- the funding system must also strengthen the links between generations and spread the financial responsibility.

Its main conclusions were as follows.

- For the UK there is no demographic time bomb as far as long-term care is concerned and therefore care will be affordable.
- The most efficient way of pooling risk, giving best value to the nation as a whole, across all generations, is through general taxation, based on need rather than wealth. This will ensure that the care needs of those who suffer from Alzheimer's disease will be recognised just as much as those with cancer.
- An hypothecated unfounded social insurance fund would not be apt for the UK. A prefunded scheme would constitute a significant lifetime burden for young people and could create an uncertain and inapt call on future consumption.
- The answer is improved state provision but only for personal care.

Its main recommendations were as follows.

- *The costs of care for those individuals who need it should be split between living costs, housing costs, and personal care. Personal care should be available after an assessment, according to need and paid from general taxation: the rest should be subject to a co-payment according to means* (Chapter 6).
- *The Government should establish a national Care Commission which will monitor longitudinal trends, including demography and spending, ensure transparency and accountability in the system, represent the interests of consumers, encourage innovation, keep under review the market for residential care, nursing care, and set national benchmarks, now and in the future* (Chapter 7).

The report was rapidly commended and strongly endorsed by the House of Commons Health Committee. The government's response was to set up a Cabinet Committee on Older People, appoint a 'Cabinet Champion' for Older People, designate the Department for Work and Pensions to take the lead on older people's issues and establish The Pension Service specifically for pensioners' benefits. As part of its approach to care planning, it created a **National Service Framework for Older People**, which has set standards for care across health and social services and involves local government, the voluntary sector and older people themselves.

Developing Effective Services For Older People (2003) GB: National Audit Office, HMSO, London.

This report accepted that the government had done the above, but recommended further actions that would in its view improve coordination, consultation, and the use of evidence in formulating policy – all issues identified in the Sutherland Report. It recommended that the planned Older People Strategy be published as soon as possible and that the Department for Work and Pensions should work to promote improvement in coordination and championship across the various government departments involved (which is most).

The overall impression, in this as in NHS policy and priority setting, is that in government documents and, recently, in practice, older people are not being ignored, indeed they are the focus of considerable central discussion and monitoring. How well this translates into local practice is, of course, a different question with different players.

Definitions used throughout government documents about the NHS

Extent and quality of services

1 **Comprehensive service** (1942): This was defined in the NHS White paper (1944) as meaning two things. Firstly, that the service was to be available to all, and secondly that it covered all necessary forms of healthcare. Necessary healthcare was also detailed (*see* p. 2) and included all conceivable healthcare needs.
2 **Reasonable requirements** (1977): This means that healthcare that is impera-tive for 'success' will be available, dependent (in this case) on the Secretary of State's sound judgement in determining what is 'within reason'.
3 **Appropriate** (1977): Healthcare provision which is considered (by the Secre-tary of State) to be suitable.
4 **Reasonable expectations** (1979): Citizens will receive the healthcare that they consider is due, if the care they want is determined to be within reason.
5 **Broad range** (1979): Healthcare of unspecified/specified (but wide) limita-tions.
6 **Acceptable** (1995): This means that the healthcare should be provided in a manner that is suitable (or just tolerable).

Access to service

1 **Equal opportunity to benefit** (1942): People have the same rights (regardless of means, age, sex or occupation) to healthcare.
2 **Equality of entitlement** (1979): To have the same rights/claim to health services.
3 **Equality of access** (1979): Same right to use the health service.
4 **Fair entitlement and access** (1991): Health services are to be provided in a just manner in terms of rights and use of healthcare.
5 **Equity** (1995): People with the same needs should receive the same standard of care.

Financial considerations within NHS principles/objectives

1 **To divorce healthcare from questions of personal means** (1944): Removal of the individual's responsibility to look after his own healthcare in financial terms.
2 **Within available resources** (1988): Not exceeding the (collective) means available.
3 **Value for money** (1988): Something worth the money spent.
4 **Priorities** (1988): The right to have healthcare before other people (cf. Access to service).
5 **Efficiency** (1995): The most effect for money spent.

Justice and solidarity with the old – two complementary moral concerns in healthcare

Mats Hansson

In a recent international project on prioritisation in healthcare it was concluded that 'Sweden may still stand out as the archetype for a society where institutionalized solidarity is very far reaching' (Bergmark, 2000, p. 408). A development of popular opinion in support of general welfare programmes indicates that governmental efforts to strengthen structures of solidarity are backed up by concerns about solidarity among Swedish citizens. Concerns about solidarity in regard to prioritisation in healthcare are also codified in national principles for prioritisation in healthcare. The proposition by the Swedish government followed from a proposal by a parliamentary committee on prioritisation in healthcare. Precedence is given to need, but palliative care and treatment of those with a low capacity for autonomy are regarded as equally important as acute care. They are, accordingly, all placed in priority group number one.

However, in a situation where real prioritisations have to be made it becomes difficult to defend a system that only meets the needs of the severely ill patients or those with a low degree of autonomy, while those with lesser but important needs will be placed on long waiting lists or will have limited access to care. This is indicated by a recent follow-up study of prioritisation in healthcare in the Swedish county councils and municipalities (SOU 2001:8, 2001). When parents cannot provide care for their children's important health needs because there are not enough doctors in the primary care units, they will not gladly vote for a system that places palliative care for the elderly in general in the first priority group. The report puts enthusiastic affirmations of the presence of concerns of solidarity in Sweden into perspective. In addition to this, reports in the mass media about maltreatment of the old at institutions for care of the elderly have become frequent during the last few years. One may suspect from this that general welfare systems based on concerns of solidarity seem to work best in times of affluence, when no real prioritisations have to be made.

Sweden is not the only country where there are indications of a decreasing concern for the old. The Royal Commissioners appointed by the Labour government in 1997 in order to examine the options for providing long-term care for the old claimed that as a society Great Britain has ceased to value old age. There have been several examples of discrimination against the old within the NHS (Ashcroft *et al.*, 2000). In this situation some are still optimistic and point, like Bergmark *et al.* (2000), to the support from public surveys. Others would like solidarity to be strengthened as the necessary infrastructure of any society committed to justice in healthcare and equality in the allocation of resources (Houtepen and Ter Meulen, 2000a). I will in this article argue that there should be room for solidarity in the construction of national systems for allocation and prioritisation in healthcare, but solidarity is then a particular kind of moral concern that should be distinguished from and complementary to concerns of justice.

Justice and solidarity at stake

When real prioritisations have to be made it is evidently not only solidarity that is at stake. Justice is a key issue in prioritisations in healthcare. However, it is important to distinguish them from each other and see that they both have a role to play in guiding moral and political decision making in the healthcare sector. Houtepen and Ter Meulen regard solidarity as 'a quality of social relations, of which just outcomes are an integral aspect' and they claim that 'one cannot have solidarity without justice, but one can have justice without solidarity' (Houtepen and Ter Meulen, 2000b, p. 336). They suggest that solidarity complies with common standards of justice. These definitions are not clear with regard to the relationship between justice and solidarity and it is not explained what is meant by saying that just outcomes are 'integral aspects' of solidarity. According to a common understanding of the concept 'solidarity' such a concern is a sufficient reason for an unequal treatment of individuals. One individual is favoured because she stands in a special kind of relationship to the person acting, for example being their child or parent. The outcome of an act of solidarity may then not be just in accordance with the common criteria of justice. The benefited individual does not receive that benefit after a balancing with the other's interests in accordance with 'need', 'contributions', 'merit', 'desert' or an effort to maximise utility. The individual is benefited as a result of a concern that is not equally distributed. A person's particular need is favoured or a particular person is favoured regardless of need. Accordingly, one can have 'solidarity without justice', as well as 'justice without solidarity'.

I will outline a distinction between justice and solidarity that helps to explain our difficulties, in a growing number of welfare societies, in finding solidarity in practice in social institutions of healthcare. I will regard concerns of justice and concerns of solidarity as different but complementary moral concerns that should both be recognised in political action to organise healthcare. The focus of my discussion is allocation of resources in healthcare with a primary interest in the special outcome for the old.

Justice and solidarity as two different kinds of moral duties

Concern with justice and concern with solidarity can both be seen as moral duties but I will suggest that the duties are different. Concerns with justice are wider in terms of who is concerned. All people or all members of a certain group, say the old, are to be treated with equal respect and consideration of their interests. The concerns are, however, more limited with regard to what is at stake, the content of the moral duty. They do not take into consideration all aspects of the particular circumstances regarding what is at stake for an individual. Concerns with solidarity, by contrast, are narrow with regard to who is concerned. There is a social basis of the concern that limits the subject of interest to particular individuals who either fulfil a proximity condition or are related to the agent for some other reason (Egonsson, 1999). However, concerns with solidarity are wider with regard to what is at stake. They are imperative concerns based on knowledge about specific needs and individual circumstances.

This distinction between justice and solidarity concerns depends on the Kantian distinction between perfect and imperfect duties. Onora O'Neill has elaborated on the distinction in a discussion about children's rights and children's lives (O'Neill, 1989, pp. 187ff.). A perfect duty makes a universal claim. It specifies completely who is bound and to whom our obligation is owed. Its claim does not depend on specific cultural or social conditions. In the case of children as in the case of the old we are obliged to refrain from abuse of them whether or not they are specifically in our charge. As in accordance with the concern with justice, we are obliged to do or to refrain from doing a certain kind of action to all who qualify on certain general criteria. It is also a question of a perfect duty when those obliged have undertaken a prior commitment and responsibility, as a human task in general, or as a part of a certain social role. The duties of those who have undertaken to care for specific individuals – nurses, doctors, teachers and parents – are perfect in kind.

In addition to this, Kant, in his *Introduction to the Metaphysics of Morals*, also develops the concept of an imperfect duty (Kant, *Einleitung*). These are the duties we owe to certain persons but not to all. The term 'imperfect' does not mean that the fulfilment of the obligation is optional, or that they as obligations have less binding force compared with the perfect ones. Imperfect duties are imperfect because they, according to Kant's treatment of practical reason, are not solely grounded in the pure will. The claims depend on specific individual or social circumstances. As in accordance with solidarity concerns they make it possible to acknowledge the love of a parent to a child as a relation of special relevance or to appreciate specific knowledge about particular needs and desires of an old family member. What is left optional by an imperfect duty is the way in which the duty is enacted and the selection of those for whom our duties are performed.

According to Kant, the duties in his ethical system cannot come in conflict with each other so that one of them would annul, in whole or part, the other. 'Duty and obligation are concepts which as such express the practical necessity of certain actions, and two conflicting rules cannot both be necessary at the same time.' A conflict of duties is inconceivable. Against this background, and with concerns with justice defined as perfect duties and concerns with solidarity as imperfect duties, justice and solidarity are to be regarded as complementary.

The limited but important role of justice in healthcare

There are several models for justice in healthcare and they are discussed in more length in the main text of this book. Within the framework of the basic distinction between justice and solidarity described here, Rawls-inspired models such as Norman Daniels's are good examples of more modest approaches to justice in healthcare (Daniels, 1985). Daniels's central argument is that health is a special kind of good because in a very fundamental way it affects our opportunity to choose our way of life during its different stages. Based on a general, Rawlsian, system of social justice Daniels argues that a principle guaranteeing fair equality of opportunity should guide the distribution of healthcare resources. In selecting a system of allocation of limited resources in healthcare any prudent individual would like to secure a reasonable opportunity range at each stage of life. He would not like to reach old age and find out that he has deprived himself of all resources in earlier years. And he would not like to miss important opportunities when he is young just in order to save resources for a later stage of life, not knowing anything about his preferences at that later stage. Daniels allows for age-relative opportunity ranges in his system, taking into consideration our different needs in different phases of life but any prudent deliberator would go for an equality of opportunity ranges across his lifespan. Just out of prudential reasons, then, we should vote for a system that saves something but not too much for later years, and we should then also make sure that there is room for changing preferences and value profiles as we live through the different stages of life. The ambition is modest but it provides a normal opportunity range to all, regardless of age.

The argument is rather similar to a recent argument by Ronald Dworkin (Dworkin, 2000, pp. 307ff.). With regard to allocation of limited resources in healthcare there is one principle that is often applied both in everyday medicine and in political decision making about priorities in healthcare. Dworkin calls it the 'rescue principle'. It 'insists that society provide such treatment whenever there is any chance, however remote, that it will save a life' (Dworkin, 2000, p. 316). Dworkin's main argument is that a prudent deliberator would reject such a principle because it does not take into consideration other important values in life besides the anticipated value of the medical treatment. He asks us to consider our willingness to forgo important values related to housing, education and economic security at earlier stages of life for the benefit of uncertain prospects of life at its latest stages. Suppose healthcare was entirely based on a private insurance scheme; no prudent individual would spend so much money on his health insurance that it will cover the costs of heroic treatment of improbable value that may prolong life only by a few months if this implies that he must forgo other important values. If nations should not spend more on healthcare than we as prudent individuals would do, then this 'prudent insurance principle' suggests that justice sets limits to what should be spent on healthcare.

To save a life is not enough. We have also to consider the content of that life. Heroic treatment of improbable value is then a violation of justice. I would not like to forgo important values as a 25-year-old person in order to ensure that I am treated as a comatose patient after a stroke, with no or little conscious relationship to life. Both decisions to treat and decisions to withdraw treatment must accordingly be carefully weighed. There may be situations in medical practice when a doctor after carefully listening to and discussing with the relatives comes to the conclusion that curative treatment should be discontinued on medical grounds. The relatives may, for various reasons, want treatment to be continued but this would be for the doctor not only against what she considers best for the patient, it would also constitute a violation of justice.

Dworkin's argument is of practical relevance since a large proportion of the cost of healthcare falls within the last six months of our lives. These six months may come early in life and so his argument is not an argument that places the old in any discriminated situation. However, it does have a bearing on spending on healthcare for the old, and in particular what kind of spending during the last stages of life. In this way it puts into perspective the argument in the Swedish parliamentary committee on priorities in healthcare which in a more unqualified sense places the old and those with low autonomy in the highest priority group. If the Swedish prioritisation scheme implies that stronger efforts should be made for non-heroic palliative treatment there is no offence of justice, in Dworkin's sense. However, if this prioritisation implies heroic treatment of improbable value the consequence of the committee's work is unjust.

The implications of Dworkin's argument must be taken with some caution. It may not be so easy to decide what is of 'improbable value' in the individual case and our value preferences may change as we pass through different phases of life. Daniels made more explicit room for a change of value preferences. A healthy 25-year-old person may find the prospects of life associated with a brain injury and living the rest of his life in a wheelchair of no value. However, we know from studies regarding quality of life that value preferences change and that it may take only five years after a car accident that has driven a young person into this kind of situation before he has re-evaluated life entirely and scores as high on all quality of life measurement scales as any healthy person (Stensman, 1985). Accordingly, judgements about what is of 'improbable value' must be made with great caution and the clear-cut cases may not be as many as we might think when it comes to real choices. However, Dworkin's main point is appreciated. Some heroic life-saving and life-prolonging treatments may as such be violations of justice.

In a community committed to equality of resources, Daniels's principle of equality of opportunities across life stages and Dworkin's prudent insurance principle suggest a limited but important moral basis for allocation of limited resources in healthcare – a just allocation. In agreement with Rawls they are concerned not with individual obligations to give to those in need but with the shaping of institutions characterised by fairness. The only duty the individual citizen has, according to Rawls's argument, is the duty to help in forming such fair institutions. In my terminology this is the limited but important ambition of perfect duties regarding the allocation of resources in healthcare. However, it is not the whole story. There should be room also for taking knowledge about particular needs and desires into consideration and also for taking advantage of the specific relationships between people that are the source of this knowledge. We need not call in solidarity for help when justice will already do the job in a way that all will accept from prudential reasons, but there should be room for concerns of solidarity as a kind of imperfect duties when justice is not enough.

Solidarity – an ideologically or socially embedded moral concern

Solidarity is sometimes described as a specific type of association between people, an association with a mutual relatedness and interdependence. Solidarity is to be recognised in welfare societies that have shaped their systems of healthcare and social security in certain ways, i.e. with a specific focus on the outcomes for the poor and needy. However, I think one should first try to recognise it as a moral concern that motivates the construction and shaping of these systems and institutions in the first place. There is an element of altruism or sacrifice associated with the concept that goes beyond both prudential concerns of justice and mutual relatedness and interdependence between donor and recipient.

Following this line of thinking, solidarity may be defined as a concern for others which includes a readiness to make sacrifices and is based on a feeling of unity among individuals. This is a subjectively-based definition. However, the definition does not grasp the capacity of a social unity to carry on and express its infrastructure of solidarity, even when there are no individuals left with the corresponding will or feeling. There are interests of solidarity with the vulnerable and the needy that have been legally recognised and institutionalised. One example is the institution of marriage where certain legal provisions are made in the interests of the children. In a similar way, so called 'welfare societies' have created infrastructures of solidarity which protect certain values when the moral motivations of the individuals are not enough to promote them. Solidarity can, then, also be defined in a more objective way as an infrastructure of social relations based on social cohesion and a social recognition of individuals.

It should be observed that concerns for the poor and needy already have a place within prudential schemes of justice. According to Rawls we do not know our lots in life behind the veil of ignorance and there are reasons for any prudent deliberator to create institutions that will include special concerns for the poor and needy. Injustices may also be accepted if they are to the benefit of the poor. Rawls's general scheme invites measures to be taken with the purpose of protecting those with diminished degrees of autonomy, as is suggested in the Swedish legislation. Concerns for affordable medicine and healthcare in less developed countries and special concern for identified individuals and groups with particular needs will, however, go beyond the concern with justice. These aspirations of solidarity are inspired by different political or religious ideologies. They do not fit entirely into the definitions of solidarity given above, since they are not necessarily based on a feeling of unity among individuals. In a historic review of the Christian-Democratic interpretation of solidarity in The Netherlands, Houtepen and Ter Meulen suggest that the religious versions of solidarity stem from the tradition of charity, and that solidarity in this context 'is asymmetrically conceived in terms of a helping relationship' (Houtepen and Ter Meulen, 2000b, p. 330). This may be an accurate historic description of the motives of solidarity within these religious traditions, but these kinds of aspirations may also be symmetric in character. It is true that altruism has been the guiding idea behind the helping behaviour practised by Christians, but vulnerability has probably played an important role as well. At least, there is biblical inspiration pointing in this direction.

In contrast to a popular interpretation of the message of the parable of the Good Samaritan, it is not primarily to do with helping those in need. The key figure in the parable is not the Samaritan but the assaulted man by the road. He is a Jew and would in accordance with the rules normally never talk to a Samaritan. Seeing a person from this ethnic group he would cross the street in order not to come near. Now he finds himself in a powerless position where he has to receive help from this person, an untouchable and a person who embodies generations of hate and mistrust between the people in the region. The message of the story is that there is a special kind of unity between people based on the experience of vulnerability and that helping behaviour should be built on such symmetrical relationships. The characteristic feature of this kind of experience is that the primary objective is not to define the position of the subject (the helping or the receiving) but to realise that the self only means something in relationship to the other (Ricoeur, 1992). We share the experience of being vulnerable, and sometimes we are in need of help. This is then a special feeling of unity, to see oneself as another, fitting well with the subjective definition above.

As with the other sources of solidarity, political and religious motives need not depend on strong degrees of personal commitment. There are bonds of social cohesion built into the structures of a society that will do the job regardless of the personal convictions of its citizens. Concern for others functions as the cement of society (Elster, 1989). It has its social significance regardless of whether it expresses anything like a genuine feeling existing in the society, or only a socially and culturally established pattern of giving and receiving. Altruism and solidarity concerns should then be promoted irrespective of moral worth and regardless of people's saintliness. The novelist Sow Fall from Senegal has illustrated how norms of altruism may work in a society (Sow Fall, 1986). In the religious society she describes, the institution of alms giving regulates every transaction in all sectors of society. A certain amount of money or specified goods must be given to the poor before a contract is entered into, a sale is completed or a marriage arranged. No wonder then that the entire social system collapses on the day when the beggars decide to go on strike. Suddenly, the poor find themselves in a fruitful bargaining position with altruism. According to Sow Fall, there is a social value in the concern for others, regardless of the moral significance of people's actions and their choice of a social system.

The role of solidarity in healthcare

According to my definitions, solidarity is not 'the infrastructure of justice' as argued by Houtepen and Ter Meulen (Houtepen and Ter Meulen, 2000b, p. 336). Solidarity and justice are different but complementary concerns where the concerns of justice are wider with regard to who is entitled to care, but the level of care is limited to what would fall within the framework of prudent choices under the scheme of a general system of justice. The outcome may be a result of applying principles such as the equal opportunity principle or the prudent insurance principle, or some other principle of a similar kind. The selection of principles of justice is not what is at issue here. Rather, it is the recognition that they all in some way or another set limits to what we, as a society committed to fairness in the allocation of resources, should spend on healthcare. Heroic treatment of improbable value is unjust and sometimes it is right to refrain from saving a life, even when we have the medical and technical capacities to do so.

However, in addition to concerns with justice I will argue that we should make room for imperfect duties, concerns with solidarity. A decision not to continue treatment of a patient suffering from a stroke may be right in accordance with what would fall within the concerns of justice. However, the question is if there should be room for actions taken by the relatives of the patient, and if society should promote this kind of action. I am not implying that we should spend resources on treatments with improbable value, but there are things we might want to do as individuals, families, friends and neighbours that do not fit within the concern with justice. I will even argue that we should empower our institutions of healthcare in order to give room for solidarity, as long as it does not violate the principles of justice.

Solidarity – the basis for special knowledge about patient needs and desires

There will always be a distance between general principles of justice and the particular, multifarious circumstances of individual patient cases. Guidelines such as the Swedish national principles for prioritisation in healthcare are not sufficient in order to decide if a particular patient should be given a particular treatment. Doctors and nurses add their professional knowledge and experience, and there is a promising Swedish experience with using ethical rounds in order to develop a more context-sensitive ethical praxis (Hansson, 2002). However, sometimes professional knowledge and experience is not enough. In order to understand what is really at stake for an individual patient, knowledge is needed about the life story of this patient, her values and particular circumstances. There is a kind of knowledge about patient needs and desires that only those attached to a patient by relationships of solidarity may be able to provide. Relatives, friends, neighbours and colleagues may have vital information about what a patient enjoys, what makes life better for them and how it can be worse. They may help the patient to exercise their expertise regarding what they want to accomplish, what they are prepared to endure and what they no longer want to continue. Accordingly, if patient needs and values are at stake, which they always are, there must be room for imperfect duties such as concerns of solidarity during the entire process of care.

Solidarity between generations

In the 1999 report of a Royal Commission examining the care of the old in Great Britain it is concluded that although the lot of older people has improved the society as a whole has ceased to value old age (Ashcroft *et al.*, 2000, pp. 387ff.). The commission found that relatives experienced a strong sense of loss of control in losing a beloved individual to a system they did not fully understand and where there was no help to meet their special needs. Even if residential homes and nursing homes provide good help for their clients, the result of early discharges from hospital care is 'social exclusion of a whole section of society' (Ashcroft *et al.*, 2000, p. 338). The question is how discrimination against older people should be remedied. Ashcroft *et al.* (2000) suggest that solidarity must be a moral principle that should be translated into political will and action. They regard solidarity as 'a property of the structure of society' even if they, in agreement with the Royal Commission, conclude that this structure is of a rather weak construction. There are two questions in relationship to this that I will explore. One is concerned with how the social exclusion of the old and the weakness of the structure of solidarity in society can be explained. The other question is concerned with what kind of political action is appropriate with regard to allocation of resources for healthcare on the basis of concerns of solidarity.

One possible explanation of the social exclusion of the old is that fundamental values regarding the ageing process that would include old people presuppose a solidarity structure that we find only, or mostly, in unities of rather strong social cohesion such as families. Solidarity between generations and a special appreciation of the old is a natural thing within families, among friends and even among neighbours. Grandmothers and grandfathers today may not play the same role in sustaining the economy of the family as they did in the past, but in most families they are still essential for helping out and sustaining family relationships, values and traditions. They may sometimes contribute to the economic security of the younger family members, but their main contribution is a support of social cohesion. Outside the family, friendship and social recognition in the neighbourhood is to a great extent based on how individuals contribute to the welfare of society as part of the workforce. At least in Western societies there is a widespread conception of the stages of ageing and a view of the old that places the productive middle aged at the top and regards old people as having gradually moved down to become those who do no more than stand in the way of younger people or are in need of care, having nothing left to contribute to life, society and welfare. It is not a modern phenomenon, as can be seen from the many past pictorial and literary representations of the stages of life.

In practice the old are taken care of by those who are committed for reasons of solidarity. The majority of all care of the old is still, even in a welfare society such as Sweden, given by the family, by friends and by neighbours (Bergmark *et al.*, 2000). The fact that informal care of the old forms the bulk of all care given to them is evidence that there is another value pattern regarding the stages of ageing and the old at play in structures based on solidarity concerns. This kind of informal care, I suggest, is based on a certain kind of value structure that is not so easy to transfer to the formal care provided within national structures of health and welfare.

In a speech in 1961, the German sociologist and historian Eugen Rosenstock-Huessy presented an opposite view to the one commonly held; that life is best in youth and that you only experience a slow, inescapable decline until nobody asks for your advice and you are only a nuisance to others (Rosenstock-Huessy, 1970). The core idea of his thinking is that it is only when you have reached maturity, that is, when you have attached yourself to others and learned (childhood), and when you have detached yourself and fought (adulthood), that you are able to lead and legislate, have the credibility to teach and instruct, the wisdom to prophesy and warn and, finally, the privilege to testate, endow and bestow. Each stage is as important as in a symphony, but we don't grow and get involved without the old, they who have learned how to survive. As survivors, they have something to tell us about how to survive, how to grow and how to mature.

Stages of survival – the symphony of life

Testator	Doubter/Despondent
Prophet/Warner	Player/Singer
Leader/Legislator	Learner/Wanderer
Sufferer/Perseverer	Reader/Conceiver
Protester/Rebel	Listener/Obeyer
Critic/Analyst	

Ashcroft *et al.* (2000) give evidence of different instances of discrimination against older people, including exclusion from health services solely on the grounds of old age. In order to come to terms with this it may be necessary to rebuild the value basis of care and concerns for the old. It is not an unrealistic hypothesis that the treatment and care of older people, including decisions about when and where to discharge from hospital care, is influenced by the basic attitudes and conceptions regarding the stages of life and the old. A different value pattern may be an incentive for a doctor to think twice before deciding to discharge a patient or where to send her. To influence the value pattern in accordance with 'the stages of survival' described by Rosenstock-Huessy may be uncontroversial, but justice sets limits also to this commendable goal. Heroic treatment of improbable value is not an alternative because we also want to have other values, related to education, housing and economic security, fulfilled. The values may be an incentive to further improve palliative treatment as one of the ingredients in ordinary institutional healthcare and services. The Swedish model for treatment and care of patients with dementia developed by Sonja Thorburn in Huddiksvall is one example of this kind (Thorburn, 1990). The treatment programme is guided by the goal of rebuilding and reinforcing a patient's confidence in his or her own mental and physical capacities. Autonomy is the goal, not the ethical limit for what may be done to a patient.

However, this kind of value structure will for natural reasons have its greatest role to play within the social contexts of families, friends, neighbours and colleagues, that is, among those people who share a common history of survival and from this experience know what is at stake for an individual member of the network. These supporting individuals may be doing what is needed without any encouragement but in order to give room for these concerns of solidarity in treatment and care in a way that is broad enough, different means of empowerment may be needed.

Empowerment for supportive care

Empowerment of patients is an intrinsic part of both curative and palliative treatment. Patient education and empowerment have long proved to be critical for successful self-management by diabetes patients. Clinical outcomes in diabetes are dependent on education programmes recognising a wide range of learning strategies and individual differences regarding self-management (Day, 2000). For coronary heart disease, patient empowerment through rehabilitation and education may be important for successful secondary prevention, provided that there is an effective communication between health professionals (Holt *et al.*, 2000). Patient empowerment strategies are also proposed for stroke patients (Clark and Forbes, 2001). The majority of research going on in this area has been concerned with patient empowerment in a rather narrow sense, focusing on the patients themselves (cf. Rodwell, 1996).

However, there are signs that patient teaching is expanding into a more comprehensive inclusion of the broader agenda of health promotion and disease prevention (Roter *et al.*, 2001). Empowerment of the structures and networks that surround patients has recently received more attention. A pilot study for assessment of the efficacy of a family-to-family-programme in the support of mentally ill patients demonstrated significantly greater family, community, and service system empowerment in addition to reduced displeasure and worry about the family member who had the mental illness (Dixon *et al.*, 2001). In a research project examining the support needs of families caring for a relative in palliative care, it was demonstrated that lack of information regarding practical resources, and methods of providing practical care and of managing medications was very problematic (Wilkes *et al.*, 2000). The information that the supporting families needed must meet individual and varying needs. Sometimes the families reported not knowing about their information needs until a crisis occurred.

These are examples of empowerment for supportive care which adds a new element in healthcare and it is something that should be a responsibility for all institutions of healthcare. Supportive care is a supplement to curative treatment and palliative care within the hospital. There is no social obligation to provide this kind of care. It is an obligation of individuals based on concerns of solidarity as imperfect duties, taking particular knowledge and values about individuals into consideration. However, there may still be a social obligation of the institutions of healthcare to empower individuals to be responsible for this kind of supportive care. According to the Ottawa Charter for Health Promotion a process of enabling is required in order to help people to increase control over and to improve their health. A fundamental premise of the Charter is that 'in order to realize their freedom and assume greater responsibility for their health, individuals may require help in the form of know-how, resources, and power to assume greater control' (Yeo, 1993). Important targets for health promotion, in addition to the health and wellbeing of the individual, are families, community support groups, colleagues at the workplace and networks in the neighbourhood. In particular with regard to situations where there is need of expert knowledge about individual needs and desires about an old person, solutions to health problems require cooperative action driven by the concerns of solidarity.

In order to enable relatives, friends, colleagues and neighbours to promote health, healthcare institutions should be designed to meet this need. Empowering a family or a colleague to care for a patient may as indicated above imply information, education and expert advice. Taking into consideration the increasing amount of complex information related to health and wellbeing available in the mass media and on the internet, an important part of the service may be to help the supporters to sort out what kind of information is relevant. Research concerning empowerment of the networks of solidarity around the patient is still in its infancy but it is a development that should be encouraged.

Conclusion

Justice and solidarity are two important and complementary moral concerns. Concerns of justice imply an appeal to equality, for example that age should not be a criterion *per se* for prioritisations in healthcare. The argument by Daniels about a fair equality of opportunity across the entire lifespan supports this conclusion and so does Dworkin's argument about the prudent insurance principle. The old are included on equal terms with the young in these schemes. However, justice also sets limits to what we should spend on healthcare. To engage in heroic treatment of improbable value is from this perspective a violation of justice, not something commendable. It is not only possible to invite relatives to a discussion about the continuation of care, as did the doctor in the example with the old woman, it is a perfect moral duty. Swedish regulation and practice are not particularly clear in this respect. It is at best an invitation to rethink the basic value structures and to help us to focus on the situation of the old. It is not a help to solve real situations of prioritisation.

Solidarity invites individual and particular concerns and needs to an extent that it is not possible to allow within the national healthcare system without violating perfect duties of equality and justice. Ordinary care, both within curative and palliative treatment, may as indicated benefit from a change of the basic value patterns. A reappraisal of the old, the survivors, may have vital and practical implications within all healthcare institutions and in particular regarding questions about when and where to discharge an old patient. However, it is within socially cohesive structures such as families, support groups, networks of friends and colleagues that we will most likely find and recognise these values. Therefore it is not surprising to find that they are already responsible for a large proportion of healthcare, even within modern welfare societies such as Sweden.

Health promotion is partly a responsibility of healthcare institutions and partly something that the individual themselves must assume responsibility for. This is the same for old and young. In order to take advantage of the special knowledge of family members, friends and other solidarity networks in society they must be empowered to fulfil their duties. These are imperfect duties of solidarity but of equal moral importance to the concern with justice. It has and should be possible for people to assume responsibility for their relatives, friends, neighbours and colleagues, provided that they are willing to pay for the care. However, society should enable them to make informed decisions regarding the care of their relative. There are many agents on the private market willing to offer expensive help and those mainly interested in profit should not be allowed to take advantage of vulnerable people acting out of genuine motives of solidarity.

Approaching challenges to solidarity – an afterword

Solidarity concerns have their place and should be promoted. However, there are new challenges to the national healthcare systems coming up, challenges that will go beyond what can be met by prudential justice schemes. It remains to be seen if there is enough solidarity around to do the job. The models for achieving justice in the allocation of scarce healthcare resources in this context share a central component in their dependence on ignorance. Since we are expected to select principles of justice without having access to vital information about our value profiles, our lots in life or conditions during the last stages of our life, it is a prudent choice to select a system with fairly general welfare provision systems with regard to who should be entitled to what within the national budget for healthcare. However, the rapidly developing area of genetic diagnosis indicates that more and more individuals and patient groups in the near future will have access to vital genetic information about their health status and genetic risks. It is true that genetic constitution plays a significant role for all people, but some conditions are more expensive to treat and live with than others. If groups of patients belonging to the less fortunate in the genetic lottery are to be entitled to healthcare in accordance with their special needs, this must come as a result not of prudent deliberation but out of concern for a special kind of solidarity. It must then be a kind of solidarity that goes beyond the traditional limits of a unity of social cohesion, challenging both prudential justice concerns and the solidarity concerns hitherto known.

Justice and the Nordic healthcare systems

Vilhjalmur Arnason

Introduction

I will first sketch the problems facing the healthcare systems in welfare societies and trace their causes. The problems, I contend, are more due to a demanding mode of thought characterised by individual rights than the fact of an ageing population. I will show that while the welfare system was decisive in fighting historical injustices, solutions based on the principle of welfare are insufficient to deal with contemporary problems. I consider three alternative modes of thought:

* the market solution
* the utilitarianism implicit in the Oregon model
* a Rawlsian notion of just healthcare.

I will argue that the last one provides the best guidelines for shaping fair healthcare obligations. I then go on to draw out the main principles of prioritisation in recent reports in the Nordic healthcare systems. I will argue that these principles seem to be in line with the Rawlsian thought of securing healthcare as a primary good for everyone, and protecting in particular the interests of the worst off. This line of reasoning is best suited to guide us in the difficult task of shaping fair social obligations in the contemporary context.

Problems facing the healthcare systems in Nordic welfare societies

Let me first attempt to sketch the nature of the problem facing our system of healthcare. Briefly the situation can be described in the following way. There is an increasing gap between the demands and needs for healthcare and our ability to pay for health services from public funds. The reasons for this situation are many. I will single out five factors which I think are most important:

* a steadily increasing range of research and treatment options
* the ruling 'technologised' ideology of the healthcare profession and of the public
* higher expectations among the public
* the population is growing older
* an individual rights-based attitude to healthcare.

The first three of these go hand in hand; as people become more aware of the growing potential supply of healthcare services due to vast advancement in the biological sciences and medical technology, they also come to expect higher levels of service, and demand that even more be done to cure illnesses and even to conquer death itself. This is perpetuated both by healthcare professionals who are trained to find technological solutions to most medical problems and by the general public which believes in this mode of thinking (Kennedy, 1983; McKeown, 1976). All of this is important and would deserve a detailed analysis and discussion which I cannot undertake here. What I find most interesting in this context, however, is the fifth factor which has to do with the public perception of justice with respect to the provision of healthcare services. The individual rights-based attitude to healthcare is a branch of modernity which is characterised by the demand that each individual should be an autonomous agent and make the decisions concerning the vital aspects of their life. When this mode of thinking is coupled both with technological thought which states that everything that can be done is to be done, and the ideology of the welfare society which tends to define individual rights to services in broad terms, it is not surprising that we have a demanding population. This, I believe, is a more serious threat to our system of healthcare than the growing population of the elderly which is mainly problematic in light of the other factors.

Healthcare needs are certainly of vital importance for individuals and they are prone to think that everyone ought to have the right to all medical treatment available. Attempts to bridge the gap between actual demand and potential supply of healthcare services, by setting limits to the public provision of healthcare, meet, therefore, with great resistance in this population. I believe that the gap between affordable and possible healthcare is bound to grow in the future and if we are to come to grips with it, we must find acceptable criteria of justice which breed solidarity rather than the atomistic mentality associated with individual rights. Before I go on to develop this thought, I will look further into the implicit theory of justice that lies at the root of our present system of healthcare.

The principle of welfare – genesis and validity

The underlying principle of socialised systems of medicine in the Nordic countries could be labelled as an egalitarian welfare principle. It is instructive in this regard to look at the first article of the Icelandic law on healthcare:

> Every citizen is to have access to the best [most perfect] health-care services that at each time is possible to provide in order to protect mental, physical and social health (Act no. 59/1983).

The intention of this law is to provide everyone with equal rights to healthcare. This right is, of course, a positive welfare right which creates duties on behalf of the state to provide each citizen, indiscriminately, with the best healthcare available at each point in time.

Historically, this has been extremely important in order to improve and equalise the life conditions of people. Only a few decades ago, the public suffered from grave injustice, partly because individuals were not secured the basic rights that we now take for granted in our welfare system. The national healthcare act was a major stepping stone towards securing that everyone in Icelandic society would be provided with the primary goods (in the Rawlsian sense) necessary for each citizen to project their own plan of life. Fortunately, there was a broad political agreement about this policy which was a major matter of justice because it guaranteed the citizens a much fairer equality of opportunity than before. At the same time it provided for social cohesion because it substantiated the notion that we are jointly responsible for one another and that we will not tolerate that someone will miss the opportunities in life because of bad luck in the natural lottery of health or because of accidents.

From this historical perspective, the egalitarian principle of right to welfare has clearly been most valuable. It is questionable, however, whether it is a fruitful guideline for the new task of setting limits to healthcare. We must also ask whether it has really brought about good health services. In order to answer that it must be evaluated according to what I call the three criteria of good healthcare:

- the economic criterion of (cost-) efficiency
- the professional criterion of quality
- the ethical criterion of justice.

I will argue that a healthcare system implicitly based on the egalitarian principle of right to welfare has to some extent failed on all accounts.

First, it is not cost-efficient. Most states are now setting limits to the ever-increasing costs of healthcare. This is not least because in a scheme of equal rights of all to the best healthcare, there are no rational limits. This could work in a situation of affluence, but it is insufficient in a situation of scarcity. We are used to thinking that progress eliminates scarcity. But it is interesting to note that in the context of healthcare, scarcity can increase along with social progress. This is because it is relative to historical possibilities each time. The problem is that the 'cost of human ingenuity applied to healthcare exceeds the capacity to pay for it' (Emson, 1991, p. 1441).[1]

Secondly, our healthcare system does not guarantee optimal quality of healthcare. Major emphasis has been on the expansion of technologised hospital care at the neglect of prevention. Therefore, it has not worked according to the major goals of healthcare, which are the protection of health and the prevention of sickness. This is a complicated issue that has various explanations. Partly the situation is created by the 'ideology' and the vision especially of the medical profession towards its subject matter. Medical doctors have become increasingly specialised in the various parts of the human body, which has enabled them to get an ever-increasing mastery over sickness, but has diverted their attention from the causes of sickness and the context of disease, therapy and recovery.[2] And this appears to be supported

---

[1] I leave out the question here how much a nation can spend on healthcare. I don't see it as a law of nature that a nation should not spend more than, for example, 10% of the national expenditure on healthcare, especially in a rich country like Iceland which spends nothing on defence. The only rule that might apply here is that a nation is not to spend so much on healthcare that it is unable to uphold other institutions, such as the education service, which are necessary to provide for equal opportunity for all citizens.

[2] This is one reason why the shaping of health policy is not to be left only to the health professionals, who are likely to substitute their individual and narrowly professional interests for the public interest.

by the public who mostly prefer to lead unhealthy lives and then be saved in hospitals when the need arises. This, however, has never been put sufficiently to a democratic test. Instead, the healthcare system seems to increase in a relatively autonomous way, driven more by the technological imperative of doing whatever is possible than by a sensible standard of good healthcare.

Thirdly, our healthcare system has not contributed well enough to fair equality of opportunity among the citizens. To mention one reason: 'The fact that we get an equal chance of being cured once ill does not compensate us for our unequal chances of becoming ill' (Daniels, 1985, p. 141). Moreover, the vision of technologised medicine threatens to discriminate among patients, giving priority to those with healthcare problems that lend themselves to technological solutions. In this way and others there is always an implicit hidden rationing and prioritising of healthcare – one that is not explicitly put forward and thrown into an open public discussion. Nevertheless, defenders of a status quo in the healthcare system often appeal to a national consensus which presumably exists in society. But this is a tacit consensus, which needs to be made explicit through a public dialogue.

It seems to me that the mode of thought that historically created a healthcare system which brought about both increased justice and solidarity may threaten both if we keep going in the same direction. As the gap increases between the public expectations and possible healthcare due to ever-increasing bio-medical knowledge and technical capacity, there will be a growing discontent among the public with the healthcare system. This will be a sense of injustice, because if there is no systematic change of policy, hidden prioritisation and rationing will continue. And this will threaten social cohesion, because people will become more anxious that they and their relatives may not get the treatment and the care that they believe they have the right to receive. Such a situation of scarcity, where there are no well-defined lines of distribution of resources and social obligations, is simply bound to lead to animosity and upheaval among the citizens.

Alternative philosophical approaches

The libertarian approach

Facing this situation, the principle of individual liberty is often appealed to. It is maintained that justice, quality and cost-efficiency in particular are not ensured except through the workings of the market. To reach this goal, health services and insurances are to be privatised, increasing the responsibility of both the citizens and the professionals. Historical experience of this model, however, has shown that:

- It is not cost-effective. Healthcare in the US is the most expensive in the world. As in the welfare system, providers of the services profit from doing as much as they can. In this way it fails even when it is measured against its own major criterion, i.e. the economic factor.
- It provides optimal quality of healthcare only for those who can afford it. It leads to a one sided emphasis on high-technology medicine at the neglect of prevention, even to the point where many people are without basic healthcare. Some receive too much, others receive far too little healthcare. This attitude breeds moral indifference and social disruption. It is also based on the

false presumption that the healthcare system is only for those presently in need. Nobody gets through life without benefiting from healthcare, which is to be seen as mutual investment and insurance for everyone.

*   It is unjust. It discriminates between people on the basis of ability to pay, which is not a relevant criterion for basic healthcare. This is remedied in softer versions of libertarianism through the notion of a 'safety net' or a decent minimum of healthcare for every one. This remedy, however, has two major shortcomings. On the one hand, it invites two different types of healthcare, one for the rich and another for the poorer population. On the other hand, it violates people's self-respect, because those caught in the safety net are put in the position of receiving healthcare in the form of charity from the other part of the population which can stand on their own feet. This adds insult to injury. This position, therefore, has no commitment to the moral point of view where every person is taken equally into account. Instead it reduces all communal relations to business or market exchange.

A major reason for the deficiency of this model is that healthcare services are not the kinds of things that are properly marketed.[3] Consumer goods are of such a kind because the market insures that people have a variety of things according to their individual preferences and desires. Healthcare services, however, have little to do with individual preferences and desires; they are designed to meet some of our basic objective needs. Healthcare needs are 'course of life needs' – those needs which people have all through their lives or at certain stages of life through which everyone must pass (*see* Daniels, 1985, p. 26). These must be distinguished from adventitious needs which are the kinds of things people need in order to realise their particular contingent projects: for example, people with particular foot problems, like flat feet, need special shoes for health reasons, while others need special shoes for particular pastimes, like mountain climbing.

The utilitarian Oregon model

In light of these shortcomings of the market alternative, it is instructive to consider a health policy that was designed in Oregon state in the US. Realising that it is impossible to meet all healthcare needs, the state authorities made the decision to implement explicit rationing of healthcare. The project is based on a few basic premises (Oestbye and Speechley, 1992):

1   All citizens ought to be entitled to the same basic level of healthcare.
2   Healthcare ought to promote health.
3   Explicit choice is fairer than hidden rationing.
4   Rationing should reflect both expert analysis and community values.

After several (60) communal meetings and the work of an expert committee, they went on to devise a list prioritising healthcare services for 709 possible treatments. For each condition, the treatment was weighed against four criteria:

*   Does it improve the quality of life?
*   Does it increase longevity?

[3] Although these are strong arguments against adopting a market model as a basis of healthcare, they need not exclude market solutions in certain aspects of the health services.

- Would everyone have equal access to the service?
- Is it efficient (providing the most benefits for the most people for a given amount of money)?

Ranked highest on the list are procedures that are the most reliable, long-lasting and cost-effective in bringing about a better quality of life to the most people. At the bottom are fatal, incurable and trivial conditions; also procedures that are 'expensive and unlikely to improve the quality of life of the patients such as infertility services, cosmetic surgery, therapy for eating disorders, sex change operations and most organ transplantations' (Oestbye and Speechley, 1992, p. 93). It is the task of the legislators to decide where the red line will be drawn on the list, i.e. which services will be publicly funded and which will not.

The Oregon plan is highly interesting and instructive in this context. It provides a good example of a consciously designed health policy which is intended to benefit the greatest number in the most economic way. Compared to the system of healthcare that is widespread in the US, where a big portion of the population (13% in 1992 when the Oregon plan was in the making) has no health insurance coverage, the Oregon system is likely to strengthen social cohesion. The major gain of the plan is that everyone is provided with basic health services, which implies, for example, that the focus is now more on prevention (such as neonatal care) that benefits everyone than on high-technology medicine with question-able benefit for the few. This means that individual lives that have been heroically saved by high-tech medicine may now be lost, while the statistical lives of the many that before were lost may now be saved.[4]

There is a problem with the Oregon plan in that its utilitarian conception of benefits ('greatest benefits for the greatest number') looks primarily at numbers and threatens certain individuals with grave injustice. The plan shows well how difficult it is to choose between preventive measures of health protection on the one hand, and health services to those in acute need on the other hand. In fact, it is misleading to describe the problem in these terms. It is a prima facie moral duty to help individuals that are in acute medical need, provided that the treatment is not futile or primarily harmful. This does not mean that everyone has a right to every operation. However, it means that it is indefensible to make a wholesale macro decision to bar people from certain kinds of important health services without taking into account the individual differences in each case. The goods and harms at stake are impossible to quantify. Moreover, before drastic rationing measures are implemented all unnecessary procedures performed in the existing system must be eliminated. According to Alain Enthoven at Stanford University, about one-third of healthcare costs could be saved if we stop doing procedures that we have no evidence will benefit the patient (Oestbye and Speechley, 1992).

On the other hand, society also has a long-ranging obligation to facilitate preventive measures. This task, however, goes far beyond the role of the healthcare system and it faces many obstacles which have roots deep into our social structure. In the long run they might reduce the need for medical services or at least improve the quality of people's lives. But in the meantime no individual,

[4] Daniels (1985) points out that, while we are prepared to devote vast resources to saving identified victims, we are much less willing to use the money more effectively to save statistical victims.

regardless of age, that is in grave medical need and has good possibilities for leading an active meaningful live must be denied treatment. That seems to be a requirement of justice – unless it conflicts with the principle of fair equality of opportunity of the members of the society.

Rawlsian justice and healthcare

In order to flesh out a mode of thought about the healthcare system which can fairly limit our access to healthcare goods and provide guidelines for social obligations in this area, I suggest that we look in the direction of Rawls's theory of justice as fairness. This is a procedural notion of justice, specifying the conditions necessary for a fair distribution of goods in society. I find it most fruitful to see this primarily as a critical idea, providing a perspective from which every real agreement or consensus in society can be criticised. We can always ask: would this arrangement of things be accepted by everyone and for everyone concerned under fair conditions? Because of this, the contractarian model is inherently more democratic than the other two.

The key idea in Rawls's contract theory is that people come to an agreement about the arrangement of social institutions under a 'veil of ignorance'. This basically means that the contractors don't know what their social position or general condition will be when the veil is lifted. This makes it necessary for them to ensure everyone's share of primary goods (rights and liberties, powers and opportunities, income and conditions for self-respect) because these goods normally have a use in everyone's rational life plan. The veil of ignorance makes it impossible to promote one's own interests without promoting those of others. In this way it represents the moral point of view where everyone's interest is equally taken into account. Rawls writes:

> The veil of ignorance insures that no one is advantaged or disadvantaged in the choice of principles by the outcome of natural chance or the contingency of social circumstances (Rawls, 1972, p. 12).

It is rather remarkable that this counter-factual agreement, which is not intended to describe anything that has taken place, lends itself quite well to the discussion of just healthcare. This is because the veil of ignorance is perfectly realistic in this sphere of life. No one can know what their healthcare needs will be next year, next month or even tomorrow for that matter. Will we be paralysed after a car accident, bed-ridden because of cancer, or demented old people when the inevitable veil of time is lifted? And if we are overly optimistic and/or biased in our own case, we can apply this to our children and parents: how will they fare in the health lottery?

Norman Daniels, who has applied Rawls's theory of justice to healthcare, (Daniels, 1985; *see also* Chapter 4 of the present work) fruitfully regards health as the normal functioning of the body, seen as a psychosomatic whole, and healthcare needs are those necessary to achieve or maintain 'species-typical normal functioning' at each point in life (Daniels, 1985, e.g. p. 26). Impairment of this functioning reduces the range of opportunity open to the individual in the course of their life. This is most often due to causes that individuals have no control over. For the most part it is determined by a natural and social lottery. This is why healthcare is primarily a matter of justice; its role is to protect an individual's share of life's opportunities.[5] On this model, therefore, healthcare rights are not primary; rather the social obligations are determined by the social agreement under fair conditions. We must not, however, read Rawls's theory too narrowly as a contract theory and regard the principles of justice as fair simply because they are chosen under a veil of ignorance. We could also put it the other way around and say that the principles of justice are chosen under a veil of ignorance because they *are* fair. Rawls writes:

> The basic intuition which underlies all my ideas and which they are systematically built around, is about society as a fair system of coopera-tion of free equals. Justice as fairness is rooted in this idea as one of the basic components of democratic culture (Rawls, 1985, p. 231).

This rootedness of justice as fairness in democratic culture shows that even the liberal contractual system of solidarity is 'founded upon a pre-contractual consensus on fundamental values' (Houtepen and Ter Meulen, 2000b, p. 333). In Hegelian terms we could say that the *Moralität* of contractors under a veil of ignorance is a normative test of values already formed in the historical *Sittlichkeit* of society. On this reading one can see the hypothetical contractors under a veil of ignorance choosing to design a solidaristic system of healthcare not simply because they are rational egoists but also because they realise the dependence of individuals upon a system of social relationships and values.

This clearly places emphasis on the joint responsibility or solidarity of the citizens, but what about individual responsibility? Some people take responsi-bility for their health, while others take great risks. Prudential contractors must seek just ways to deal with this. And since they know the general facts of life, they will know how difficult it is to determine what exactly is due to voluntary decisions and what is the result of natural and social conditions. Therefore, they will not take the risk of adding injustice to injury, that is blaming the victim by discriminating between patients once the damage is done. They will rather look for indirect ways, especially through redistribution of profit from unhealthy consumption and risk activities, such as smoking and mountain climbing. Besides, they will probably want to provide themselves with some elbowroom to live dangerously, without having to pay specifically for it when they find themselves in need.[6] However, if and when healthcare needs can without doubt be shown to be voluntarily caused, it is a matter of justice that special health fees be placed on such behaviour in order to distribute the burden of healthcare costs fairly (Veatch, 1981, Chapter 11).

What kind of health policy would hypothetical contractors design under a veil of ignorance? Rawls has not tried to address this question but according to Daniels, it is likely that if we were to construct a system of healthcare under a veil of ignorance we would agree that:

- Everyone should have equal access to services needed to maintain, restore and replace a person's normal functioning and to protect the fair share of opportunities in the course of his/her life.

---

[5] The normal opportunity range for a given society is the array of life plans reasonable persons in it are likely to construct for themselves (Daniels, 1985, p. 33).

[6] This may be more a humanitarian reason than a requirement of justice.

- They would prefer a scheme which would enhance a person's chance of reaching a normal lifespan to a scheme which reduced the chance of reaching a normal lifespan, but giving those reaching a normal lifespan an increased chance of living longer.
- They would put emphasis on providing healthcare services which maintain an active meaningful life but not merely on prolonging it.
- They would want the system to protect an individual's share of the normal opportunity range by reducing the risks of disease and disability, by seeking an equitable distribution of the risk of disease (e.g. by work safety regulations), and by curing disease when it arises (in this order).
- In general they will find it more important to prevent, cure or compensate for those disease conditions which involve a greater curtailment of an individual's share of the normal opportunity range than to treat those conditions that affect it less.
- It is not a social obligation to provide health services which arise from individual preferences and are not necessary to restore a person's normal functioning.

These points do not imply any specific suggestions for rationing or prioritising healthcare services. Instead, they are indicative of the mode of thought that needs to be strengthened in our task of reconstructing the healthcare system. This means, for example, that we give up the one-sided emphasis on healthcare on demand, backed by individual rights, and try to reach a consensus on social obligations to provide quality care which is both just and cost-effective. In dealing with the macro-allocation of healthcare goods and the making of general health policy, it is most necessary to form a social agreement about general principles. Such a consensus requires broad public discussion which ensures that people take responsibility for the policy made, and identify with it. This was properly attempted in the Oregon project, but nevertheless it suffers from a serious flaw which shows that democratic discussion is not sufficient to reach a fair consensus. The discussion must also be enlightened by a proper notion of justice.

Here we must keep in mind that a major concern of justice is to provide equality of opportunity. In the context of healthcare this means removing the hindrances that limit people's opportunity range and result from injury, sickness or disability, or increase their chance of suffering from these conditions. Rawls argues convincingly that under a veil of ignorance primary goods would be distributed equally unless an unequal distribution of these goods is to the advantage of the worst off. And the 'worst off' in this context are those in greatest medical need, that is those who suffer from conditions that threaten to radically reduce their share of the normal opportunity range. This can for example be the case with many organ transplantations which in the Oregon plan are unfairly ranked with cosmetic surgery and sex change operations at the bottom of the list. This is indicative of the moral problem in the Oregon project. Robert Veatch has argued that throughout the process the focus was on identifying which care was basic, not which care was fair to provide (Veatch, 1991). This does not mean, however, that everyone should have the right to organ transplantations. Since the important issue is to distribute healthcare goods fairly over an individual's life, age is clearly a relevant factor. A life-saving organ transplantation can be an obvious requirement of justice when young people are concerned, but may be far less so when people have already lived most of their natural lifespan. The situation is quite different with conditions such as infertility services, cosmetic surgery and sex change operations which can hardly be called grave medical needs. There are options for these people other than medical operations. We may know some individuals that would like these services and we may have sympathy for them. That is one reason why the veil of ignorance is important for these kinds of decisions. It makes us unable to know the individual identity of the contractors (as we can never know exactly which health services people might need in the future). This is one of the reasons why the goddess of justice is blindfolded.

The acceptance of these limits may be the major social obligation of each individual – a mark of solidarity and citizenship. It also requires that we will not continue to be slaves to medical technology, but that we subordinate it humbly to the appropriate ends of medicine (Callahan, 1987, p. 173). In fleshing out the idea of a social consensus on healthcare, we are bound to move from the unlimited individual rights-based attitude to just general rules which set limits to healthcare that everyone can in principle accept, and which guide the shaping of social obligations. The result of such a contract might not be entirely different from the Nordic socialised medicine we know, but I believe that it will provide us with more sensible and more explicit guidelines to make healthcare more efficient, professional and just.

Nordic plans of prioritisation

The problems mentioned at the start as threatening our healthcare system have increased the need to forge a health policy. This implies that decisions have to be made about prioritisation of the tasks of the healthcare system. A successful prioritisation is a way to secure that everyone can have a necessary healthcare service when the need arises, that money is effectively used and that professional criteria are employed in order to define and demarcate the healthcare services that should be financed by the state. Such a health policy, therefore, would meet the ethical criterion of justice, the economic criterion of (cost-) efficiency and the professional criterion of quality. Clearly, a successful prioritisation is a matter of justice, because it requires that policy decisions are made according to publicly available criteria which can be openly debated and assessed. Otherwise, the prioritisation is arbitrary, concealed and subject to private interests.

In recent years, the Nordic nations have systematically undertaken the task of pondering the criteria of fair prioritisation in healthcare. Although the conclusions are of various types, it is nevertheless possible to discern the key common aspects.[7] In fact, there is not so much dispute about the ethical standards which I will now try to briefly summarise.

The principle of human dignity or equal respect

It is not surprising that this principle is the foundation of any West European reasoning about just healthcare. The idea of moral equality of all citizens is

---

[7] I have in mind the following reports: *Priority-setting in the Health Service* (Denmark, 1996); *From Values to Choices* (Finland, 1995); *Priorities in Health Care* (Sweden, 1995). There is an English summary in the Icelandic report *Forgangsroedun ì heilbrigdismalum* (1998).

literally undisputed in the moral and political philosophy of our time, although there are disagreements about how best to observe it (e.g. *see* Kymlicka, 1990, p. 4). The minimal requirement it implies is that healthcare must not discriminate between people and that patients shall receive similar treatment for comparable illnesses, independent of social status, age, income or other accidental factors. This also implies that people shall have equal access to healthcare services, regardless of where they happen to live in the country.

The principle of solidarity

As mentioned above, this is one of the main characteristics of the ethics of the welfare society. Solidarity implies that individuals are not only responsible for themselves but also co-responsible for their fellow citizens (Houtepen and Ter Meulen, 2000a). In practice, this makes itself manifest in the fact that healthcare is publicly financed but not merely by those individuals who use the services on any particular occasion. Thus everyone lives in the security that they can seek medical aid when they need it regardless of their ability to pay. It can be said that the principle 'from each according to ability, to each according to need'[8] is the backbone of this principle of solidarity. Special emphasis is placed on securing the healthcare of those groups of people who have a weak standing due to age or handicap.

It has been argued that the (European) principle of solidarity is quite different from the (American) liberal principle of justice (Houtepen and Ter Meulen, 2000b). I have my doubts about that. It seems to me that Rawls's contract theory reconciles the individual motivation to protect one's interests with the requirement to secure social reciprocity protected by institutions. Rawls could, therefore, in his own way, accept Habermas's idea that justice and solidarity are two sides of the same coin:

> Morality cannot protect the one without the other. It cannot protect the rights of the individual without also protecting the well-being of the community to which he belongs (Habermas, 1989, p. 200).

Habermas has the explicit dialogical emphasis which makes his theory a more fruitful candidate than Rawls's for constructing a notion of a democratic, discursive solidarity which is sorely needed in the reappraisal of our system of healthcare. In spite of the lack of dialogical condition in the Rawlsian theory, however, we should be mindful of the fact that the function of the veil of ignorance is not only to make the contractors ignorant of their own position but also to make them more knowledgeable about the human condition in general and about various individual situations. As a theoretical exercise it inspires us to imagine ourselves in the situation of the worst off and thus it motivates our vision of interdependence and reciprocity in human relations. It can thus function as a 'reflexive solidarity' as described by Houtepen and Ter Meulen which implies 'continuous reappraisal of the way that institutions and services affect the people involved in caring practices' (Houtepen and Ter Meulen, 2000a, p. 373). This, I believe, is for example made manifest in a strong sense of solidarity in Norman Daniels's theory of just healthcare.

[8] Marx's famous dictum from the *Critique of the Gotha Programme*.

The principle of medical need

This principle is already implied in the principle of solidarity as it is understood in the Nordic prioritisation reports. Healthcare needs are of various sorts and it is a matter of justice that those who have the gravest healthcare needs should have priority.[9] The problem is, of course, to determine which are 'the gravest health-care needs' and to find out what is comparable in that regard. Most recommendations about prioritisation in healthcare imply ideas about which services are to be emphasised above others. In the Icelandic report it says, for example:

> Priority shall be based on need for healthcare. The following services and forms of treatment shall have priority.
> 1   Treatment of acute or life-threatening illnesses, physical or mental, and injuries which can lead to serious disability or death.
> 2   Preventive healthcare, which has proved effective.
>   The treatment of serious long-term illnesses.
>   Rehabilitation and habilitation.
>   Palliative terminal care.
> 3   Treatment of less serious injuries, and acute and long-term illnesses of a less serious nature.
> 4   Other forms of treatment which professional experience has shown to be effective.

Cost-effectiveness

This principle urges healthcare professionals to choose the less expensive option of any two that have the same effectiveness. The notion of effectiveness refers here to the benefit that an individual can receive from a particular treatment. When many people need the same treatment, it can also be a matter of justice to choose the less expensive option, even though the benefits are somewhat less for each individual, because in that way effectiveness can be increased (Swedish Government Report, 1995, p. 107). Futile treatment should not be provided, nor expensive treatment which has a high sacrifice cost.

Individual responsibility

In contemporary society, illnesses are increasingly related to lifestyle for which individuals can be said to be, at least partly, responsible. This appeal to responsibility does not mean that individuals will be charged for healthcare services, but rather that preventive medicine and health promotion need to be planned in the light of this fact. Moreover, some problems are such that individuals can better deal with them than the healthcare system.

---

[9] Matthews distinguishes desires and needs and argues that people have a legitimate claim to have their needs met (Matthews, 1998, pp. 156–7).

Conclusion

I think that it can be fairly concluded from this that the Nordic countries are determined to maintain their principles of justice and solidarity in the face of the rapidly changing situations of society. They have neither succumbed to the libertarian demand of privatisation of healthcare nor to the utilitarian calculations of benefits. Instead, their moral principles of prioritisation seem to be in line with the Rawlsian thought of securing healthcare as a primary good for everyone, and protecting in particular the interests of the worst off. The historical agreement about justice as solidarity has been strengthened in the social dialogue that has taken place. Although official reports are words that need to be substantiated by policies and actions, they are nevertheless important indicators of the self-understanding of the citizens in this regard. They are in fact crucial now when there is an increased admittance of the fact that unlimited application of the welfare principle can overthrow the healthcare system. In such situations, our adherence to equality is put to the test because we can no longer escape the task of finding out which inequalities are justifiable and which are not. The aim of a just welfare system is to contribute to the eradication of unjust inequalities. The healthcare system does this by maintaining and restoring the normal functioning of individuals so as to enable them to have a fair share in life opportunities. It is a matter of justice to remove obstacles due to illness and injuries that hinder people in realising this objective and to shape the social obligations in light of it. This, I believe, is a much more fruitful approach than referring to the indiscriminate rights of individuals to healthcare.

References

Aaron HJ and Schwartz WB (1984) *The Painful Prescription: rationing hospital care* (Brookings Studies in Social Economics). The Brookings Institution, Washington DC.

Abelson J (2001) Understanding the role of contextual influences on local health care decision making: case study results from Ontario, Canada. *Social Science and Medicine.* **53**(6): 779–93.

Alamowitch S, Eliasziw M, Algra A, Meldrum H *et al.* (2001) Risk, causes, and prevention of ischaemic stroke in elderly patients with symptomatic internal-carotid-artery stenosis. North American Symptomatic Carotid Endarterectomy Trial (NASCET) Group. *The Lancet.* **357**: 1154–60.

Ashcroft RE, Campbell AV and Jones S (2000) Solidarity, society and the Welfare State in the United Kingdom. *Health Care Analysis.* **8**: 377–94.

Austin D and Russell EM (2003) Is there ageism in oncology? *Scottish Medical Journal.* **48**(1): 17–20.

Battin MP (1994) *The Least Worst Death*: essays in bioethics at the end of life. Oxford University Press, New York and Oxford.

Bebbington AC (1988) The expectation of life without disability in England and Wales. *Social Science and Medicine.* **27**(4): 321–6.

Bergmark Å (2000) Solidarity in Swedish Welfare – standing the test of time? *Health Care Analysis.* **8**: 395–411.

Bergmark Å, Parker MG and Thorslund M (2000) Priorities in care and services for elderly people: a path without guidelines? *Journal of Medical Ethics.* **26**: 312–18.

Beveridge Report (1966) *Social Insurance and Allied Services.* Report by Sir William Beveridge, presented to Parliament November 1942. Cmnd. 6404. HMSO, London.

Blaikie A (1999) *Ageing and Popular Culture.* Cambridge University Press, Cambridge.

Bowling A (1999) Ageism in cardiology. *British Medical Journal.* **319**: 1353–5.

Braybrooke D (1968) Let needs diminish that preferences may prosper. In: N Rescher (ed.) *Studies in Moral Philosophy.* American Philosophical Quarterly Monograph Series, No. I. Basil Blackwell, Oxford.

Brody B (1989) Towards quantifying the health of the elderly. *American Journal of Public Health.* **79**(6): 685–6.

Butler J (1999) *The Ethics of Health Care Rationing.* Cassell, London and New York.

Butterworth S (2001) *A study into the extent of changing trends in disability status and their potential effect upon health services utilisation in the UK.* MSc Dissertation, Department of Public Health, University of Aberdeen.

Callahan D (1987) *Setting Limits: medical goals in an aging society*, Simon & Schuster, New York and London.

Callahan D (1990) *What Kind of Life: the limits of medical progress*, Simon & Schuster, New York and London.

Callahan D (1995) Aging and the life cycle: a moral norm? In: D Callahan, RHJ Ter Meulen and E Topinková (eds) *A World Growing Old: the coming health care challenges.* Georgetown University Press, Washington DC, pp. 20–27.

Cassel CK (1999) The Limits of Setting Limits, reprinted in JD Arras and B Steinbock (eds) *Ethical Issues in Modern Medicine* (5e). Mayfield Publishing Co., Mountain View, California, London and Toronto, pp. 658–62. (Originally published in P Horner and M Holstein (eds) *The Limits of Setting Limits.* Simon and Schuster, New York.)

Cassel CK and Neugarten BL (1994) The Goals of Medicine in an Aging Society, reprinted in T Beauchamp and L Walters (eds) *Contemporary Issues in Bioethics* (4e). Wadsworth Publishing Co., Belmont, California, pp. 93–102. (Originally published in 1991 in: RH Binstock and SG Post (eds) *Too Old for Health Care? Controversies in Medicine, Law, Economics, and Ethics*. Johns Hopkins University Press, Baltimore, MD.

Clark WR (1999) *A Means to an End: the biological basis of aging and death*. Oxford University Press, New York.

Clark D and Forbes C (2001) Patient empowerment in stroke – a strategy for Scotland. *Scottish Medical Journal*. **46**(3): 71–2.

Community Care and Health (Scotland) Act 2002. The Stationery Office, Edinburgh.

Coulter A and Ham C (2000) *The Global Challenge of Health Care Rationing*. Open University Press, Buckingham.

Cox BD, Huppert FA and Whichelow MJ (1993) *The Health and Lifestyle Survey: seven years on*. Dartmouth Publication Co., Aldershot.

Daniels N (1985) *Just Health Care*. Cambridge University Press, New York.

Daniels N (1988) *Am I My Parents' Keeper?* Cambridge University Press, Cambridge.

Daniels N and Sabin J (1997) Limits to health care: fair procedures, democratic deliberation, and the legitimacy problem for insurers. *Philosophy and Public Affairs*. **26**: 303–50.

Danish Report (1996) *Priority-setting in the Health Service*. The Danish Council of Ethics, Copenhagen.

Day JL (2000) Diabetic patient education: determinants of success. *Diabetes/Metabolism Research and Reviews*. **16**(Issue S1): 70–4.

Dean J (1995) Reflective solidarity. *Constellations*. **2**: 114–40.

Dixon L, Stewart B, Burland J, Delahanty J *et al.* (2001) Pilot study of the effectiveness of the family-to-family education program. *Psychiatry Services*. **52**(7): 965–7.

Dworkin R (2000) *Sovereign Virtue: the theory and practice of equality*. Harvard University Press, Cambridge MA.

Egonsson D (1999) Local solidarity. *Ethical Theory and Moral Practice*. **2**: 149–63.

Elster J (1989) *The Cement of Society: a study of social order*. Cambridge University Press, Cambridge.

Emson HE (1991) Down the Oregon trail. Rationing the Oregon way: the way for Canada? *Canadian Medical Association Journal*. 145.

Eraker SA and Politser P (1994) How decisions are reached: physician and patient. In: J Dowie and A Elstein *Professional Judgement: a reader in clinical decision-making*. Cambridge University Press, Cambridge.

Finnish Government Report (1995) *From Values to Choice*. STAKES, Helsinki.

Fried C (1978) *Right and Wrong*. Harvard University Press, Cambridge, MA.

Fries JF (1983) The compression of morbidity. *Milbank Memorial Fund Quarterly – Health and Society*. **61**(3): 397–419.

Frith L (1999) Priority setting and evidence based purchasing. *Health Care Analysis*. **7**: 139–51.

Giddens A (1994) *Beyond Left and Right*. Polity, Cambridge.

Gillon R (1985) *Philosophical Medical Ethics*. Wiley, Chichester.

Grimley Evans J (1997) Rationing health care by age: the case against. In: B New (ed.) *Rationing: talk and action in health care*. King's Fund and BMJ Publishing, London. pp. 115–21.

Habermas J (1989) Morality and ethical life: does Hegel's critique of Kant apply to discourse ethics? In: *Moral Consciousness and Communicative Action*. Polity Press, Cambridge.

Hanlon P, Walsh D, Whyte BW, Scott SN *et al.* (2000) The link between major risk factors and important categories of admission in an ageing cohort. *Journal of Public Health Medicine*. **22**(1): 81–9.

Hansson MG (2002) Imaginative ethics – bringing ethical praxis into sharper relief. *Medicine, Health Care and Philosophy*. **5**: 33–42.

Harris J (1988) More and better justice. In: JM Bell and S Mendus (eds) *Philosophy and Medical Welfare*. Cambridge University Press, Cambridge. pp. 75–96.

HM Treasury (2002) *Government Expenditure on Public Services: how taxpayers' money is spent. Appendix 1 of Public Expenditure Report*. www.hmtreasury.gov.uk accessed 19/08/02.

Hoffmeyr U and McCarthy TR (1994) *Financing Health Care*. Kluwer Academic Publishers, Dordrecht.

Holt N, Johnson A and de Belder M (2000) Patient empowerment in secondary prevention of coronary heart disease. *The Lancet*. **365** (9226): 314.

Houtepen R and Ter Meulen R (2000a) Solidarity in health care. *Health Care Analysis*. **8**: Special issue.

Houtepen R and Ter Meulen R (2000b) New types of solidarity in the European Welfare State. *Health Care Analysis*. **8**: 329–40.

Hunter DJ (1997) *Desperately Seeking Solutions: rationing health care*. Longman, London. pp. 97–114.

Icelandic Government Report (1998) Forgangsroedun í heilbrigdismalum. The Ministry of Health, Reykjavik.

INVOLVE (2004) *Involving the public in NHS, public health, and social care research: Briefing Notes for Researchers*. Second edition. www.invo.org.uk accessed 29/06/04.

Irvine B, Green D, McKee M, Dixon A and Mossalios E (2002) For and against: social insurance – the right way forward for health care in the United Kingdom? *British Medical Journal*. **325**: 488–90.

Kant I (1911) Einleitung in die Metaphysik der Sitten, Kants gesammelte Schriften, Königliche Preussche Akademie der Wissenschaften. Berlin: G Reimer, **IV**: 224.

Kelly S and Baker A (2000) Healthy Life Expectancy in Great Britain, 1980–96, and its use as an indicator in United Kingdom Government strategies. *Health Statistics Quarterly*. **7**: 32–7.

Kendrick S and Conway M (2003) *Increasing emergency inpatient admissions among older people in Scotland: a whole systems account*. Whole System Project Working Paper No 1. Scotland, ISD.

Kennedy I (1983) *The Unmasking of Medicine*. Paladin, London.

Kirkwood T (2001) *The End of Age: why everything about aging is changing*. The BBC in association with Profile Books, Ltd., London.

Kneeshaw J (1997) What does the public think about rationing? A review of the evidence. In: B New (ed.) *Rationing: talk and action in health care*. King's Fund and BMJ Publishing, London.

Kymlicka W (1990) *Contemporary Political Philosophy*. Oxford University Press, Oxford.

Lancet (2003) Editorial. The coming crisis of long-term care. *The Lancet*. **361**(9371): 1755.

Levitt R, Wall A and Appleby J (1999) *The Reorganised National Health Service* (6e). Stanley Thornes, Cheltenham.

Light D and Hughes D (2002) A sociological perspective on rationing: power, rhetoric and situated practice. In: D Hughes and D Light. *Rationing: constructed realities and professional practices*. Blackwell, Boston, MA.

Manton K and Gu X (2001) Changes in the prevalence of chronic disability in the United States black and non-black population above age 65 from 1982 to 1999. *Proceedings of National Academy of Sciences*. **98**(11): 6354–9.

Matthews E (1998) Is health care a need? *Medicine, Health Care and Philosophy*. **1**: 155–61.

Maynard A, Bloor K and Freemantle N (2004) Challenges for the National Institute For Clinical Excellence. *British Medical Journal*. **329**: 227–9.

Mays N (2000) Legitimate decision-making: the Achilles' heel of solidaristic health care systems. *Journal of Health Services Research and Policy*. **5**(2): 122–6.

McKeown T (1976) *The Role of Medicine*. The Nuffield Provincial Hospitals Trust, London.

McNamee P, Gregson B, Buck D, Bamford CH *et al*. (1999) Costs of formal care for frail older people in England: the resource implications study of the MRC cognitive function and ageing study. *Social Science and Medicine.* **48**: 331–41.

National Statistics (2002) *General Household Survey.* National Statistics. The Stationery Office, London.

New B (1998) The rationing agenda in the NHS. In: B New (ed.) *Rationing: talk and action in health care.* King's Fund and BMJ Publishing, London.

NHS and Community Care Act 1990 (1989) HMSO, London.

NICE Citizens' Council 2004. *Report on age.* www.nice.org.uk accessed 24/03/04.

O'Neill O (1989) *Constructions of Reason: explorations of Kant's practical philosophy.* Cambridge University Press, Cambridge.

Obermann K (2000) *Public Participation in the Rationing of Health Care.* Shaker Verlag. Aachen.

Oestbye T and Speechley M (1992) The Oregon Formula: A better method of allocating health care resources. *Nordisk Medicin.* **107**: 92–5.

Overall C (2003) *Aging, Death, and Human Longevity: a philosophical inquiry.* University of California Press, Berkeley, Los Angeles and London.

Personal Social Services Statistics (2002a) www.doh.gov.uk/HPSSS/TableE5 accessed 29/08/02.

Personal Social Services Statistics (2002b) www.doh.gov.uk/HPSSS/TableC5/6 accessed 14/09/02.

Polder J, Bonneux L, Meerding WJ and van der Maas PJ (2002) Age-specific increases in health care costs. *European Journal of Public Health.* **12**: 57–62.

Public Accounts Committee (2003) *Ensuring the effective discharge of older patients from NHS acute hospitals.* Thirty-third report. The Stationery Office, London.

Rawlins MD and Culyer AJ (2004) National Institute for Clinical Excellence and its value judgements. *British Medical Journal.* **329**: 224–7.

Rawls J (1972) *A Theory of Justice.* Oxford University Press, Oxford.

Rawls J (1973) *A Theory of Justice* (first paperback edition). Oxford University Press, Oxford and New York.

Rawls J (1985) Justice as fairness: political not metaphysical. *Philosophy and Public Affairs.* **14**: 223–51.

Rawls J (2000) Justice as Fairness, reprinted in RC Solomon and MC Murphy (eds) *What is Justice? Classic and contemporary readings* (2e). Oxford University Press, New York and Oxford, pp. 281–6. (Originally appeared in *Philosophical Review.* **67**. 1958.)

RAWP (1976) *Department of Health and Social Security Resource Allocation Working Party: Sharing Resources for Health in England (RAWP Report).* HMSO, London.

Ricoeur P (1992) *Oneself as Another.* The University of Chicago Press, Chicago.

Rodwell CM (1996) An analysis of the concept of empowerment. *Journal of Advanced Nursing.* **23**: 305–11.

Rosenstock-Huessy E (1970) *I am an Impure Thinker.* Argo Books, Inc., Norwich.

Roter DL, Stashefsky-Margalit R and Rudd R (2001) Current perspectives on patient education in the US. *Patient Education and Counseling.* **44**(Issue 1): 79–86.

Royal College of Physicians of London (1995) *Setting Priorities in the NHS.* Royal College of Physicians of London, London.

Sabin JE and Daniels N (2002) Managing disappointment in health care: three stories from the USA. In: B New and J Neuburger (eds) *Hidden Assets: values and decision-making in the NHS.* King's Fund, London. pp. 141–56.

Seshmani M and Gray A (2002) The impact of ageing on expenditures in the National Health Service. *Age and Ageing.* **31**: 287–94.

Shegog RFA (1981) *The Impending Crisis of Old Age: a challenge to ingenuity.* Published for the Nuffield Provincial Hospitals Trust. Oxford University Press, Oxford.

Solomon RC and Murphy MC (2000) *What is Justice? Classical and contemporary readings* (2e). Oxford University Press, New York and Oxford.

SOU 2001:8 (2001) *Prioriteringar i vården. Perspektiv för politiker, profession och medborgare.* Slutbetänkande från Prioriteringsdelegationen, Stockholm, p. 14.

Sow Fall A (1986) *The Beggars' Strike* or *The Dregs of Society.* African Classics. Longman, Harlow. (Original: La grève des bàttu. Les Nouvelles Editions Africaines du Sénégal 1979.)

Spillman BC and Lubitz J (2000) The effect of longevity on spending for acute and long-term care. *New England Journal of Medicine.* **342**: 1409–15.

Stearns SC and Butterworth S (2001) *Demand for, and Utilisation of, Personal Care Services for the Elderly.* Health and Community Care Research Findings No.7. Scottish Executive Central Research Unit, Edinburgh.

Stensman R (1985) Severely mobility-disabled people assess the quality of their lives. *Scandinavian Journal of Rehabilitation Medicine.* **17**: 87–99.

Sutherland S (1999) (Chair) *With Respect to Old Age: long term care – rights and responsibilities.* A Report by the Royal Commission on Long-Term Care. Cm. 4192-I. The Stationery Office, London.

Swedish Government Report (1995) Swedish Parliamentary Priorities Commission. *Priorities in Health Care: ethics, economics and implementation.* Swedish Government Official Reports 1995: 5. Fritzes, Stockholm.

Thorburn S (1990) Människovärde och människosyn ur en långvårdsläkares perspektiv. In: S-O Andersson, *Lidandet och makten.* Gothia, pp. 53–8.

UK Health Statistics (2001) *United Kingdom Health Statistics. 2001 edition.* National Statistics UKHS No. 1. The Stationery Office, London.

Veatch RM (1981) *A Theory of Medical Ethics.* Basic Books, New York.

Veatch RM (1991) Should basic care get priority? Doubts about rationing the Oregon way. *Kennedy Institute of Ethics Journal.* **1**(3): 187–206.

Wanless D (2001) *Securing Our Future Health: taking a long-term view.* Interim report. HM Treasury, London.

Wanless D (2002) *Securing Our Future Health: taking a long-term view.* Final report. HM Treasury, London.

Wellard (2000) *Wellard's NHS Handbook 2000/01* (15e). JMH Publishing, East Sussex.

Wilkes L, White K and O'Riordan L (2000) Empowerment through information: supporting rural families of oncology patients in palliative care. *Australian Journal of Rural Health.* **8**(1): 41–6.

Williams R (1990) *A Protestant Legacy.* Clarendon Press, Oxford.

Williams A (1997) Rationing health care by age: the case for, and Rejoinder to John Grimley Evans. In: B New (ed.) *Rationing: talk and action in health care.* The King's Fund and BMJ Publishing, London. pp. 108–13 and pp. 121–3.

Yeo M (1993) Toward an ethic of empowerment for health promotion. *Health Promotion International.* **8**(3): 225–35.

Index